Health Advocacy for Minority Ethnic Londoners

Putting services on the map?

Mike Silvera

Rukshana Kapasi

King's Fund

NHS Executive London

Published by
King's Fund Publishing
11–13 Cavendish Square
London W1G 0AN

First published 2000

ISBN 1 85717 435 6

A CIP catalogue record for this book is available from the British Library

Available from:

King's Fund Bookshop
11–13 Cavendish Square
London
W1G 0AN

Tel: 020 7307 2591
Fax: 020 7307 2801

Printed and bound in Great Britain

Cover photogpaphs: Robert Aberman, Minuche Mazumdar Farrar, www.JohnBirdsall.co.uk

Contents

Appendices

Acknowledgements

We wish to acknowledge the support of a wide range of organisations across London, who supplied us with details of local agencies to assist the mapping exercise.

We also wish to thank those agencies that participated in the study and provided further help in arranging focus group discussions with people who use their services.

In particular, we would like to thank all the service users who took part in the focus group discussions and shared with us their rich and valuable experiences.

Last, we thank the Project Reference Group, who met with us regularly to discuss the research project and the issues emerging from the study. They played a vital role in helping to distil and refine and number of the many complex areas emerging from this study. Members of the Reference Group were:

Jonathon Coe	Westminster Mental Health Advocacy
Naaz Coker	Race & Diversity Director – King's Fund
Susan Elizabeth	Grants Director – King's Fund
Yohannes Fassil	Community Liaison & Development Manager – KCW Health Authority
Anjum Fareed	London Ethnic Health Network – London Regional Office
Nolliag Frost	Training & Development Manager – Citizen Advocacy Information and Training
Anne Jensen	Making Training Work
Steve Gillam	Programme Director, Primary Care – King's Fund

Minara Karim	Ethnic Services Manager – Barking Havering & Brentford NHS Trust
Farida Malik	Health Advocacy Service Manager – Newham General Hospital
Sarah Mudd	Project Co-ordinator – Barts and London NHS Trust
Misak Ohanian	Centre for Armenian Information & Advice
Pushpa Sisangia	Linkworker Manager – Barnet General Hospital
Winston Trew	Faculty of Health – South Bank University

SILKAP Consultants is a health and social care consultancy formed by Rukshana Kapasi and Mike Silvera. SILKAP has stimulated pioneering work at the 'vanguard of change' in the equality arena over the last decade. SILKAP combines a passion for equality with a fundamental belief that all its work should have a practical application and value in changing service delivery, organisation and the 'experience' of the user. Most recently, SILKAP's portfolio has included Sick of Being Excluded *(for the ALG, 2000) and the production of national guidelines for ethnicity monitoring in primary care.*

Foreword

The issue of health advocacy for minority communities is central to the King's Fund's concerns with health inequalities and promoting cultural diversity and equality of access to health care.

This report, commissioned from SILKAP, is the first-ever attempt to map the little-understood interface between NHS services and users and patients from minority ethnic communities.

As the report vividly demonstrates, health advocates in minority communities undertake a range of roles and activities. These may include interpreting, information provision, health education, advocating for people's rights, local research into health needs, community development and informal mental health counselling. Health advocacy emerges as a thriving activity with 163 separate organisations around London providing information about their services. Services exist for almost every ethnic group in the 1991 Census categories, through levels of provision vary substantially, both by target communities and geographically around London.

Many advocates are highly skilled individuals (advocates will often be fluent in more than one minority language as well as English, have highly developed interpersonal skills, and practical skills ranging from counselling to health promotion work). Users of health services place high value on advocacy services, in helping them understand health services and their rights to treatment, and in tackling the prejudice and racism they encounter in their lives.

Yet the research also makes it clear that health advocacy remains a marginalised and under-valued activity. With no recognised qualification or accredited training for health advocates, advocates' work occupies a low status in relation to other health or social care professionals. Funding for services is patchy and highly insecure, often coming from charitable trusts or from funding 'pots' outside mainstream NHS budgets.

The challenge ahead is to bring health advocacy into the mainstream. The policy environment has rarely been more conducive to action: the Macpherson report into the death of Stephen Lawrence has put tackling institutional racism on the agenda in the public sector, while the Government's social exclusion agenda is underpinning a raft of new initiatives in urban regeneration. The London Health Strategy, launched by the London Regional Office of the

NHS, identifies the health of minority ethnic communities as a key priority. The National Plan for the NHS commits the service to becoming patient-centred and to the establishment of patient advocate and liaison services in every NHS trust.

To take advantage of these opportunities, the King's Fund, as part of its Millennium Grants programmes, has set aside £1 million to invest in key areas highlighted by this report:

- building networks and partnerships among providers and commissioners of services
- developing quality standards for the provision of health advocacy services
- developing accredited training for health advocates.

We will be working to build recognition that advocacy is not an optional extra but an essential tool in improving the health of some of London's most disadvantaged communities.

Susan Elizabeth
Director of Grants

Executive summary

Over a quarter of London's population is from black and minority ethnic communities. The huge diversity among different cultural and ethnic groups has presented a significant challenge for the provision of accessible and appropriate health and social care. Demographic changes, such as the growing minority ethnic elderly population and the increasing number of refugees and asylum seekers, challenge our health and social care systems, which still have much progress to make towards becoming fairer, equitable and more accessible to minority ethnic communities.

The socio-economic impact of poverty and deprivation is much more severe for London's minority ethnic communities and their health than for the white indigenous communities. One London health authority found that over half of its new cases of tuberculosis were among people who had arrived in the UK fairly recently. Additionally, many refugees have physical and psychological health needs associated with traumas experienced in their countries of origin.

Barriers to mainstream health and social care services include a complex array of poorly organised and delivered services, inadequate communication services for non-English speaking groups, direct staff insensitivity to users' cultural and religious needs, and institutionalised barriers that perpetuate discriminatory behaviour and poor practices.

This study was commissioned by the King's Fund and the London NHS Region to map the range and scope of health advocacy providers for black and minority ethnic communities across London, and to develop a clearer understanding about how the effectiveness of such services could be assessed. The study aimed to provide valuable baseline information on which strategic investment decisions could be made regarding options to support and develop health advocacy services and health advocates themselves.

Our study defined advocacy as helping people to say what they want, obtain their rights, represent their interests and gain the services they need. The fundamental emphasis of advocacy is that it sees things from the service users' perspective and recognises that the user or patient is in an unequal power relationship with the service provider. Advocates who work with black and minority ethnic users very often relay not only cultural, religious, language and social messages about clients to professionals but also, where necessary, challenge discrimination and racism. Understanding the different ways in which such a complex spectrum of activities can effectively improve access and choice is an important step towards defining the best ways to enhance the role of health advocates and improve their skills.

The method

Four groups were defined as sources of information for the study: users of advocacy services, organisations that provide advocacy services, organisations that fund advocacy services, and organisations that provide training for advocacy workers. A questionnaire was designed for each group of agencies and mailed through lists that were compiled by contacting local umbrella and 'link' organisations in each health authority and local authority borough. Users were contacted through the advocacy agencies that returned a questionnaire and invited to participate in a focus group discussion.

The total number of questionnaires returned included 163 advocacy agencies, 19 funding agencies and eight training agencies. One-hundred-and-fifty-two users participated in the focus group discussions.

Health advocacy for black and minority ethnic communities in London

We grouped the agencies in our sample as '*advocacy providers'* (whose *main* job is providing advocacy) and '*generic providers*' (those who provide advocacy as *part of their general services*). Advocacy providers comprised just over a quarter of the survey sample. The majority of advocacy and generic providers are based in the voluntary sector with a handful located in the statutory sector. All the statutory-based advocacy providers were based in NHS trusts.

Generic providers received their funding from a more diverse range of sources than advocacy providers (which were often funded by one or two agencies). There was a wide disparity among the generic providers, for example a third of these agencies provided services without any direct funding for doing so, and many of the services they offered were to support clients to use NHS services in hospitals and the primary care sector.

The study identified that advocacy is provided as a core service by many agencies working with black and minority ethnic communities. Many communities rely on small, partially funded groups to provide advice and assistance when using health and social care services. However, the capacity of smaller agencies to respond to the needs presented by their clients is severely restricted by limited resources for service provision and development.

On average, agencies had just over four paid members of staff, with generic providers relying on the involvement of unpaid voluntary staff to a much greater degree than advocacy providers. The majority of black and minority ethnic agencies fell into the category of generic provider. Not surprisingly, we found that the more established minority ethnic communities were better served by local agencies than the more recently arrived refugee communities. African and Bangladeshi communities received the highest coverage by all agencies. In many instances it was not possible to identify where specific groups were targeted, as many agencies used blanket terms such as 'African', 'Asian' or 'Eastern European' to indicate the groups they worked with. Nevertheless, certain groups such as Somalis received a much higher proportion of services than any other refugee group of equivalent size, based on the statistics available to us. This is significant, as there are many other groups of similar size in London for which there were very few 'specific' services indicated, such as Armenians (for which only one group was identified). Overall, more than half of the sample were black and minority ethnic organisations and were generic providers. The main thrust of the advocacy support they provide is to assist people to gain access and articulate their needs.

Mental health, children and families, young people, older people and people with HIV/AIDS fell into the top coverage for advocacy and generic providers. While this pattern may be indicative of levels of need, other factors such as access to funding and development resources also need to be taken into account.

The pattern of advocacy provision by many agencies highlighted the fact that links and relationships with the statutory agencies they were assisting clients to use were in many cases quite poor. Advocacy providers that were based within NHS organisations had, as would be expected, good local links within their parent organisation, as they were regarded as part of the services provided by the trust. However, few others reported good all round links. Many non-statutory advocacy providers stated that it was difficult to establish good working relationships with their statutory 'partners'. They spent enormous amounts of time and energy on managing relationships – time and energy that could be better spent on providing and developing services.

Generic providers tended to have links with a wider range of agencies and most appeared to be associated with a local network of voluntary groups or advocacy agencies. The exception was the smaller agencies, of three or less paid staff, which identified that they had poor or no links with any local networks. An apparent weakness in the links identified by all agencies was with Community Health Councils and Racial Equality Councils. Poor links were also highlighted with the primary care sector generally. However, it should be noted that the research took place when primary care groups were being set up and would not have had the infrastructure in place to reflect the types of links anticipated.

Users' perspectives

One-hundred-and-fifty-two users participated in 15 focus group sessions held as part of the study. The majority of users were contacted through agencies that had returned a questionnaire.

Everyone who participated in the focus groups acknowledged a need for advocacy support. This was described in terms of getting help to understand basic rights and entitlements to services, help to obtain ongoing support to make the most effective use of services, help to deal with discrimination and prejudice, and help to learn skills to cope in a new environment.

Users were unanimous in their perceptions that the advocacy support they received helped them to feel more confident about using services and, consequently, get more out of the service. Refugees and asylum seekers and people whose first language was not English were among those with the most immediate and pressing needs for advocacy support. Many recent arrivals, in particular some Eastern Europeans, did not have established communities in the UK that they could turn to for social and moral support, and indicated that they had experienced hostility and intolerance from individuals within the local communities in which they were placed. The holistic advocacy support provided by community organisations was critical for these groups. Many users pointed out that black and minority ethnic community organisations were often in a unique position to support them in dealing with racism and discrimination.

User expectations were quite high and certainly required advocates to have a broad knowledge of statutory and local voluntary sector services, well-developed communication and negotiation skills, and a high level of personal confidence.

Most people wanted a service that would be available when they needed it. Many people who had long-term illnesses indicated that support was often not available at the times when they were most vulnerable, at nights and during weekends. There was consensus that an advocate should be able to work with them in any situation or with any of the services that they used; their health, housing and social care needs were inextricably linked. Users also wanted to maintain continuity of contact with their advocate so that they could build their confidence and reduce their dependence as part of an ongoing relationship.

Key themes from the research

Mainstreaming advocacy

Many agencies felt that advocacy should be a 'core' element of delivering services in a city such as London, which has such wide diversity and disadvantage. There was a strong belief that advocacy services lacked investment and were not recognised or valued sufficiently within health and social care settings. Reasons included a low value associated with user empowerment and choice, limited awareness of and commitment to advocacy among many managers and professionals, and the lack of empirical evidence about the added value and cost benefits that advocacy may offer. These problems were compounded by the fact that people who tend to use advocacy services are among the most vulnerable and discriminated-against groups in society. There was a perception that some professionals often resented the role of the advocate, seeing it as interfering, threatening or unnecessary – a view that did not help in promoting the development and use of advocacy services. However, this perception is balanced by very positive views expressed by some doctors who have welcomed the involvement of advocates.

Strategic co-ordination and improved networking

The majority of advocacy providers highlighted the need to develop a dedicated network that would promote the growth and strategic development of health advocacy services for black and minority ethnic communities, promote the sharing of good practice and learning, and raise awareness and promote a more acceptable image of advocacy across health and social care sectors. They felt that the lack of such a mechanism contributed to fragmentation and poor sharing of information. Such a development, if pursued, would need to be properly funded and supported within the NHS.

Monitoring and standards

Advocacy providers stated that they had few objective measures in place to assess the effectiveness or impact of their services. Many agreed that developing objective criteria would help to create more consistency and raise standards, as well as enhancing the status of advocacy agencies. However, while seeing the value of 'core standards', some agencies saw a danger in trying to professionalise advocacy, which could be counter-productive and jeopardise many smaller agencies that often target very vulnerable groups. One of the outcomes of this study has been the production of a framework describing key features that funding bodies and advocacy agencies can adopt to assess effectiveness.

Independent advocacy or not?

It was apparent that different advocacy organisations, while practising in a similar fashion, held different understandings of the nature and principles underpinning advocacy. The key dilemma was whether advocacy services should be completely independent of mainstream service providers or whether they could operate just as effectively within larger organisations.

The 'non-independent' (statutory-based) agencies pointed to clear advantages that working as part of the NHS afforded, such as developing easier working relationships by being part of the mainstream service and having more secure funding. Ironically, these were some of the main practical concerns of independent agencies (voluntary sector-based).

Most voluntary agencies felt that the principle of independence was important for the integrity of the service. Others did not feel as strongly and argued that it was important not to take up polarised positions in this debate.

While the debate continues, we feel it should be unbiased and open to all perspectives. The litmus test should be whether the service is meeting the needs of the users it was established for. At present, there appears to be scope and a need for a range of approaches that can appropriately serve the needs of the many different communities in London.

Developing small providers

There are a large proportion of small black and minority ethnic agencies that provide invaluable support to local communities. Their ability to grow and develop and provide a high quality service is questionable when a large number of them operate with very few or no funded staff. These groups need targeted assistance and development support to raise them to a level where they can begin to participate more effectively and compete more fairly. Funding agencies offered similar views that smaller agencies should receive infrastructure development.

Primary care issues

Many providers highlighted huge areas of unmet need in primary care, particularly within GP practices. Common experiences were of GPs refusing to use advocacy and interpreting services and not understanding the needs of refugees and asylum seekers. Some providers indicated that the barriers they experienced in primary care were not confined to the use of advocacy services but reflected fundamental inequalities in service delivery.

Funding issues

The sourcing and availability of funding for advocacy services was a concern for most agencies. The majority of black and minority ethnic agencies receive short-term funding, making it difficult to achieve any significant impact or real growth and development. In addition, many of these agencies lack the support needed to produce competitive applications and find it difficult to develop their services as they wish to, because of short-term funding.

There was a strong view that funding programmes should be monitored and evaluated and feedback provided to communities about the improvements that result from their funding programmes.

A number of funders recognised the need to develop longer-term funding for voluntary sector organisations. Some acknowledged that the lack of safeguards made it easy to cut the funding of small voluntary sector organisations rather than other projects. While some expressed a need for collaboration to achieve longer-term funding, those who had tried had experienced difficulties working together to agree common standards and sustainable funding.

Training issues

There is a limited range of training available for health advocates. Much of what does exist is associated with dedicated schemes or services and therefore is not widely accessible. Even less is available for bi-lingual advocates who will often work as interpreters as well as advocates. Many agencies agree that this is an area that needs clearer and more widely acknowledged role definitions in order for services and training to be developed further and in a more strategic way.

Advocacy and training providers felt strongly that training for health advocates should be linked to a career structure. To achieve this, it would be necessary to establish links with prospective employers to provide incentives and employment opportunities. However, the level of interest and involvement of employers within health and social care agencies is very limited.

Bi-lingual health advocacy training must address both the interpreting and advocacy skills of the learner. In many of the courses available, learners could sometimes only pursue one of these options due to resource constraints.

Many training courses are heavily influenced by funders' priorities, which do not always match those of the training providers. There is no current standardisation of advocacy training across London, although training providers recognise the need for a common standard. The options that can be pursued to achieve accredited standards include the Open College system, the National Professional Qualification Body or the National Vocational Qualification.

Moving forward

Progress will always be slow if isolated and disjointed initiatives continue to be the norm. More effective action can be taken through mobilising the expertise and voices of all advocacy services in campaigning, raising awareness, training and developing and improving services. The National Plan for the new NHS promotes fast, fair and convenient services for patients. Central Government encourages user empowerment and choice across all public sector services. There are now key opportunities to promote advocacy among statutory service agencies. These include national policy initiatives such as Best Value, Quality Protects, Sure Start, Social Inclusion and many NHS programmes, like Healthy Living Centres, Health Action Zones, Health Improvement Programmes and clinical governance. All of these present some scope and opportunity to raise awareness of and standards about the way in which advocacy can be developed and utilised within the statutory sector.

The key areas for development that emerged from the study include:

- improving the funding and commissioning of advocacy
- building capacity among advocacy providers
- policy development and research
- developing standards
- developing and supporting easier access to standardised accredited training
- strengthening networking and partnerships.

1. The context and methods

1.1 Introduction

London is the most ethnically diverse of all UK cities. Recent London Research Centre estimates[1] show that about 25 per cent of London's population are from black and minority ethnic groups. Within individual boroughs the proportion of the local population from minority ethnic groups ranges from 5 to 45 per cent. The largest communities come from the Indian Sub–continent, Africa, the Caribbean and Ireland. In the 1991 Census every borough recorded at least one ethnic community of more than 2000 people, with many boroughs having seven or eight groups.[*, 2] Appendix 1 provides a more detailed breakdown of London's black and minority ethnic groups.

Statistics from the London Research Centre show that among many black and minority ethnic groups, people over 65 will increase by 100–200 per cent over the next 15 years.[3]

The majority of statistics available on deprivation indicate that black and minority ethnic groups are over-represented against indicators such as employment, housing, income level and incidence of long-term limiting illness. The socio-economic impact of poverty and deprivation is much more severe for London's minority ethnic communities and their health. Some of the statistics are alarming. For example:

- in 1995, unemployment for 16–24 year old non-white groups was 40 per cent, compared to 17 per cent in white groups[4]
- the household income profile in London shows that black and minority ethnic groups form the largest percentage of households on the lowest income[5]
- black and minority ethnic people are disproportionately represented in poor housing in London[6]
- about 180,000 black and minority ethnic households are in 'housing need', based on levels of overcrowding, sharing and children living above the ground floor[7]
- black children and Irish children had higher rates of long-term illness than any other ethnic group[8]

---

[*] These statistics took no account of other ethnic groups such as Turks and Orthodox Jews.

- Bangladeshi adults aged 30–34 had nearly twice the rate of long-term illness than white people of that age.[8]

A growing number of refugees and asylum seekers are settling in London. In some London boroughs refugee populations are in the order of 15,000–20,000. Overall, they constitute 5 to 8 per cent of the Greater London population. One study of refugees in the UK[9] suggested that 85 per cent of refugees in the UK live in London.

Refugees are among the most vulnerable groups in the capital and many have existing health problems that need addressing. Research in 1997 by East London and City Health Authority found that over half the Authority's new cases of tuberculosis were among people who had arrived in the UK fairly recently.[10] Many refugees have health needs associated with atrocities endured in their countries of origin, such as physical trauma (the after effects of torture) and mental health problems, including post-traumatic stress disorder (PTSD).

Local evidence reveals, for example, that:

- in Haringey 51 per cent of refugees who responded to the research had been tortured/imprisoned[11]
- out of 100 survivors of torture referred to psychiatrists in London, 42 had a 'major depressive disorder', 55 received diagnoses of depression and 54 of PTSD[12]
- in Brent & Harrow a survey of 573 individuals showed that self-reported mental health problems were over five times higher among refugees than non-refugees[13]
- in Newham a survey of 1151 refugees found that 44 per cent of men and 25 per cent of women said they were depressed[14]
- a Home Office survey found that two-thirds of the sample reported high levels of distress and that 83 per cent 'did not feel part of the community'.[15]

More broadly, minority populations have a higher incidence of certain conditions, such as diabetes, coronary heart disease, stroke and thalassaemia.[16, 17] In London, almost half of all mental health admissions are people from minority ethnic communities or those who were not born in the UK. In spite of poor ethnic monitoring, service uptake data shows that minority ethnic groups, and especially those of African Caribbean origin, are over-represented among patients who are 'compulsorily detained' and are under-represented among those who use 'talking therapies'.[18]

Barriers in access to mainstream health and social care services are exacerbated by problems of language and poorly provided service information. Medical professionals may lack the training, skills or access to appropriate health promotion materials to deal sensitively with issues such as female genital mutilation and its gynaecological consequences, or with mental health issues, which may be highly stigmatised in many refugee communities.

However, barriers to the access and use of services by minority ethnic groups go beyond the existence of language difficulties or staff insensitivity. The impact of socio-economic disadvantage and discrimination on the health and well-being of black and minority ethnic Londoners is illustrated by data collected in *The Fourth National Survey of Ethnic Minority and White People Living in England and Wales.*[19] This survey showed significant independent relationships between the reporting of 'fair' or 'poor' health and 'perceived racial discrimination', 'experienced racial harassment' and 'socio-economic disadvantage'.[†]

1.2 Why is action needed now? Central Government imperatives

In the wake of the Macpherson Report,[20] the enquiry into the death of the London teenager Stephen Lawrence, there is now explicit acknowledgement of the existence of institutional racism in British society as:

> *... the collective failure of an organisation to provide an appropriate and professional service to people because of their colour, culture or ethnic origin. It can be seen or detected in processes, attitudes and behaviour which amount to discrimination through unwitting prejudice, ignorance, thoughtlessness, and racist stereotyping which disadvantage minority ethnic people.*

[†] *The Fourth National Survey of Ethnic Minority and White People Living in England and Wales* showed that:

- manual workers had a 60 per cent greater chance of reporting fair or poor health than those in non-manual occupations
- people reporting experiences of racially motivated verbal abuse had a 50 per cent greater chance of reporting fair or poor health than those who had not experienced racial harassment
- people reporting experiences of racially motivated assault or damage to their property were over twice as likely to report fair or poor health.

The report has also stimulated a more concentrated focus and activity in many public sector institutions to address the effects and impact of racism because as Macpherson concludes:

> *If racism is to be eliminated from our society there must be a co-ordinated effort to prevent its growth.*

Providing culturally sensitive and competent services are a central part of the Government's programme to reduce social exclusion and inequalities in society at large. The health of minority ethnic groups is recognised as an important marker for measuring success in improving the health of the population in general.[21]

This 'political will' is mirrored by strategic initiatives from central Government, which attempt to deliberately shift the focus for tackling equality from disjointed initiatives to core strategic priorities for local government.

For example, key Government policy papers[22–25] stress the need to reduce inequalities in health and social care and to ensure that there are no disadvantages in terms of access to services. The Department of the Environment, Transport and the Regions' Best Value programme[26] has specified a comprehensive set of performance indicators to drive the agenda for local authorities. The majority of the Best Value performance indicators specify 'fair access' among their core standards. These link closely with other central Government policy initiatives, such as Agenda 21,[27] which focuses on regenerating local communities and building the capacity of local organisations.

1.3 Local London opportunities

In London there has been a raft of initiatives highlighting the shortcomings of health and social care services in meeting the needs of minority ethnic communities, refugees and asylum seekers. More importantly, these have also identified real opportunities for change. Publications such as *Addressing black and minority ethnic health in London – A review and recommendations* by the London Regional Office,[28] the work of the Health of Londoners project in *Refugee Health in London* and, most recently, the launch of *Sick of being Excluded*, a report by the Association of London Government, all highlight a range of basic changes 'needed to ensure that black and minority ethnic people are not excluded from getting the services they are entitled to'.[29] The London Health Strategy, launched by the London Regional Office,[30] identifies the health of black and minority ethnic people and refugees and asylum seekers as a key priority in working to improve the health of Londoners. The opportunities identified by all these initiatives provide a range of actions that commissioners and providers of health and social care services can take to develop solutions and change the existing status quo of inequality in service provision.

1.4 What is health advocacy?

Advocacy is about helping people say what they want, obtain their rights, represent their interests and gain the services they need.[‡] The fundamental emphasis and focus of advocacy is that it sees things from service users' perspective and recognises that a user or patient is in an unequal power relationship with the service provider. As White and colleagues[31] point out, advocates working for black and minority ethnic clients often relay not only linguistic, but also cultural, religious and social messages about clients to professionals and, where necessary, challenge discrimination and racism.

It is important in a study of this nature to distinguish between the roles of advocates and interpreters, as it is often assumed that language provision is all that is required to make services to black and minority ethnic communities accessible. Further, reviews of interpreting and linkworker schemes across health and social services[32] highlight the fact that while many of these schemes were developed to address communication difficulties, many have needed to extend their remit to include 'advocacy' roles of promoting better health and making health care systems more accessible.

Fulop and Jewkes[33] describe the role of an interpreter as 'someone who finds out from the patient the answers to the staff's questions and relays to the patient the staff's wishes or directive. An advocate's role is the opposite – to find out from the staff answers to the patient's questions and communicate their wishes.' While this description is simplistic and does not sufficiently reflect the reality of what interpreters often do, it does capture the essence of the key difference between an interpreter and an advocate. An advocate:

---

‡ From the definition used by Westminster Advocacy Service for Senior Residents.

- puts the needs, wishes and interests of the service user first
- works to clearer and more defined outcomes, with the aim of helping the service user to achieve their rights and obtain the very best from services
- is proactive in meeting the needs of the service user
- often provides services across boundaries and may not be confined to one interaction with a specific service provider.

The key role of an interpreter, on the other hand, is to be impartial in any communication or negotiation; it is not to represent the interests of either party in the communication as his/her role is to 'encode' messages and information from the service provider to the service user and vice-versa. The interpreter often provides a specific service that is confined to communicating with a service provider and user at a specific point in time.

1.5 The role of black and minority ethnic groups in providing health advocacy

The manner in which many black and minority ethnic groups work readily slots them into an 'advocacy role'. In many instances this is their *raison d'être*, as is borne out by much of the research carried out within black and minority ethnic voluntary groups.[§] An exercise of this nature needs to recognise the breadth of services that exist within the black and minority ethnic voluntary sector, beyond those that are provided directly or partially by NHS bodies. For example, there are NHS funded advocacy initiatives established to work with black and minority ethnic communities, which employ 'health advocates'. Many of these services define their role entirely within an NHS context. There are also a vast range of voluntary agencies working with black and minority ethnic groups that may provide similar services on a smaller scale but across a much wider spectrum of the health and social care sector.

Health advocates in minority communities embrace a range of roles and activities. These include interpreting, information provision, health education, advocating for people's rights, local research into health needs, community development and informal mental health counselling. Their effectiveness depends on the personal skills of individuals. Individuals in

---

[§] See, e.g. Silvera M. *Another Way to Empower People: Advocacy Research Project, Report*. London: KCW Health Authority, 1998; SILKAP Consultants Ltd. *Home Care for Black and Minority Ethnic Communities in Leeds, Leeds Involvement Project.* Leeds: SILKAP Consultants Ltd, 1998; SILKAP Consultants Ltd. *Feasibility Research: of Black and Minority Ethnic Carers, Cultural Unity Working Group*. London: SILKAP Consultants Ltd, 1998.

these roles will have a range of titles, such as 'linkworker', 'advocate', 'bi-lingual worker', 'bi-cultural worker', 'lay health worker' and 'community health worker', to name a few.

Understanding the different ways in which such a broad spectrum of advocacy activities have evolved and operate is important in defining how best to utilise the richness and diversity of such services in developing future services within the health sector.

1.6 The development and funding of health advocacy services

A number of reviews have highlighted the variability in the provision of advocacy services throughout the NHS and also the variability in the training that advocates receive. This is reflected in user experiences of advocacy services; the most comprehensive review to date, of 712 users from minority ethnic communities, revealed that advocacy practices seem to vary considerably – as do the interpersonal communication skills of advocates.[34]

In terms of funding, as with the funding of black voluntary sector organisations,[**, 35] the funding of health advocacy services in London is often on a short-term, 'soft money' basis. This has resulted in marginalised status, lack of sustainability of initiatives and a lack of investment in building the essential infrastructures of organisations. Criteria for securing core long-term funding is increasingly based on service agreements, performance management and monitoring measures.

1.7 The specific health and social care needs of refugee communities

Local work and research in London[36] has shown that black and minority ethnic users complain about poor access and negative experiences of health and social care services more than their white counterparts. Problems are compounded for refugees and asylum seekers,

---

** *Healthy Relationships*, the first substantive study to look at the support provided to the voluntary sector since the major NHS reforms of the 1990s, indicated that black and minority ethnic agencies received about 2.9 per cent of total spending in the sector. Any analysis can only conclude that this spending is far too low. In fact, the study proposed that consideration should be given to increasing investment for BME agencies in the sector to more closely represent the black and minority ethnic population in London, which stands at approximately 25 per cent.

who are often most vulnerable, as one Brent resident highlighted during a recent local consultation exercise:

> *As a refugee, you feel more vulnerable and you live with the feeling that you have no rights.*[37]

This may result in inappropriate use of secondary care services as refugees are unable to access community services and primary care. For example, the use of some A&E services, such as St Mary's in Paddington, seems to be higher among refugees than in the general population.[38]

Basic access to primary care services through GPs is a major issue for refugees and asylum seekers in London. There is a now a growing – and alarming – body of evidence that highlights the fact that refugees and asylum seekers still encounter basic problems when registering with GPs. For example, an Islington study found that 38 per cent of refugees encountered problems registering with a GP,[39] and work in Brixton and Lambeth, Southwark and Lewisham found that some patients are asked for passports when trying to register.[40]

There is also growing evidence that refugees in London experience poor access to services and numerous communication difficulties, which often results in them becoming isolated from mainstream health and welfare services.[41] For example:

- 43 per cent of the Haringey sample and 53 per cent of respondents in Brent & Harrow stated they needed an interpreter when seeing a GP. Language was also cited as a key barrier to access in Brixton[42]
- a feeling that professionals may not understand their problems and a lack of cultural understanding were cited by respondents in the Home Office Survey and the Haringey work as to why refugees and asylum seekers had not sought help for their problems[43]
- some boroughs have explicitly identified that African refugees suffer from discrimination, racial abuse, unemployment and isolation due to a perceived high prevalence of HIV among their communities[44]
- in Newham, 93 per cent of survey respondents said they had been given no information on how to register with a GP and 97 per cent said they had been given no information on how to use hospital services.[45]

The barriers to accessing equitable health and social care have certainly been made worse recently with the introduction and phased implementation of the Immigration and Asylum Act 1999. The interim 'dispersal' scheme introduced in December 1999 in London and the South East to alleviate accommodation shortages is likely to mean that refugees and asylum seekers are relocated on the basis of available housing alone, without regard to whether the area has an existing minority ethnic population that could help new arrivals to access voluntary and community support. This is likely to result in greater isolation for many people and a high level of consequent stress, because boroughs outside of London and in other major cities have less well-developed services and community support networks to meet the needs of refugees and asylum seekers. It is clear that access to advocacy is essential when the evidence shows that many refugees and asylum seekers do not receive even their basic entitlement to services.

1.8 Scope of the mapping exercise

We were very conscious of the wide range and often confusing and contradictory definitions used within the field to describe a number of related activities. We know, for example, that 'advocacy' is sometimes used interchangeably with 'bi-lingual interpreting'. While those who use the terms in this way may understand their meanings as they use them, it is harder and more confusing for those who need to make use of these services to assume correct meanings in the absence of clear-cut distinctions. As the available training in this field is not standardised, many trained health advocates see their roles and responsibilities differently.

To develop a 'working definition', we examined some of the commonly associated activities and roles identified in this area, in relation to black and minority ethnic communities in general and to the NHS in particular. Appendix 2 highlights these roles and also the definitions of advocacy we took into account in deriving our definition of advocacy for this mapping exercise.

To overcome the problems of different definitions of advocacy (and in some cases a lack of definition) among our target audience we agreed the definition below to clarify the activities that advocates may perform to help respondents select whether or not the study was relevant to their work.

Advocates are people, paid or unpaid, who speak up for and support the wishes of another person. Advocacy is about helping people to:

- say what they want
- obtain their rights
- represent their interests
- gain the services and practical support they need.

For the purposes of this study we use the term *'health advocacy'* to include the following activities:

- helping people to say what their health needs and problems are
- helping people obtain their rights to health care from GPs, hospitals, hospices, mental health services, dentists, health visitors, community nursing services, etc.
- representing a person's interest to any agency or individual in the health care system
- ensuring people obtain the services and practical support they need to ensure they or their dependants are as healthy as they can be.

Health Advocacy can take place in many settings: in *hospitals*, in *GP surgeries*, in *community services or organisations*. Health advocates may be *paid* or *unpaid*, and can have a range of titles. Some of the most common are *'health advocate'*, *'linkworker'*, *'bi-lingual worker'* or even *'interpreter'*.

1.9 Aims of the mapping exercise

The objectives of the study were to produce:

1. A list of *health advocacy* initiatives across London, with details of their target communities, funding sources, structure and links with other initiatives
2. A listing of the type of training available for health advocates in London
3. Examples of best practice in health advocacy work
4. An analysis showing the scale of health advocacy provision within each health authority, across London as a whole and for significant minority groups

5. An analysis showing respondents' views on the effectiveness of health advocacy work, future priorities in the development of health advocacy work, the factors influencing funding activity by statutory and charitable funders, and observable links with other initiatives

1.10 Methods of the mapping exercise

To ensure that we had focused and comprehensive coverage within the project timeframe, we used the following methods to collect data and respondents' views on the key issues:

Method	*Relevance to outputs and outcomes*
1. Questionnaires	• Baseline data on range, scope, structure and funding of advocacy provision • Baseline data on advocacy training provision
2. Focus groups	• Views on effectiveness, good practice and future developments, models of providers and funders • Services users' views of quality, accessibility, usefulness
3. Reference group	• A forum with valuable expertise, whose opinions would enhance discussion and debate on key issues (e.g. views on effectiveness, good practice and future developments) relating to the research process and findings and final recommendations
4. In-depth interviews	• Views of funding bodies on issues affecting funding • Exploration of exceptional issues that may emerge • Views on effectiveness, good practice and future developments
5. Telephone interviews	• For follow-up for new/additional contacts made to enhance response rate

Appendix 3 provides a detailed summary of whom we targeted across London and the methods we used to achieve our aims.

The methods identified above were determined by a number of factors.

First, the King's Fund and the NHS London Regional Office were keen to complete the study within a six-month timescale. This necessitated using an approach that would elicit fairly quick responses while, at the same time, encouraging as broad as possible an uptake.

Second, there was no current baseline from which to work. Thus, we had no comparator to aim for and only vague indicators of the number of agencies who were health advocacy providers. While we were aware of some specific health advocacy organisations, we expected to capture a much broader range of organisations because we assumed that many agencies would provide advocacy of one sort of another without necessarily describing it as such; by describing the activities they undertook, these could be placed within a wider definition of advocacy. This was an important starting point as we expected that many black and minority ethnic agencies would fall within this category. It was therefore important to capture these agencies to provide a representative picture.

This assumption created a difficulty, as we had to trawl very broadly, thereby running the risk of trying to include every voluntary agency. We therefore produced a working definition of health advocacy for the study from a literature review of relevant work, as mentioned earlier. The definition described a range of activities that agencies commonly undertake on 'health advocacy', and was provided as part of the information pack sent out with the questionnaires as well as being included on the questionnaires themselves. Agencies were asked to identify themselves on the questionnaire as either a main advocacy provider or not.

This approach enabled us to achieve the wide trawl we aimed for, as well as allowing agencies to select for themselves whether they felt the questionnaire was relevant to their work. The drawback was that this necessitated a very wide initial trawl of organisations to allow self-selection to be made by potential respondents. Again, because of the time constraints, we had to assemble mailing lists for local agencies as quickly as possible. This very much relied on the good will of local agencies and the availability of local information. Both these considerations created difficulties in obtaining local lists and agreeing who should be targeted. After our initial deadline we agreed to extend the timescale, send out a second, more targeted mailing using a list of agencies that had responded to the survey thus far. This was sent to the original contact agencies, asking them to check whether our list mirrored all the local agencies they expected to see on it and, where possible, to provide additional contact details of missing groups. This proved to be a useful approach as it increased the final response rate by 20 per cent (the responses increased from 134 to 163).

1.11 The project reference group

A Project Reference Group (see Appendix 4 for the list of members) was set up as an important part of the process of this study. The Group comprised individuals working in provider, training and funding organisations. It met every six weeks and acted in an advisory, 'think tank' capacity for the duration of the study. Group members shared valuable expertise and opinions in structured discussion groups and debates on the key issues being examined in the study, such as *effectiveness*, *good practice* and *future developments*, as well as on the research process, the findings and final recommendations. The Group also discussed opportunities and threats presented by wider changes and suggested ways in which the project could benefit.

An important outcome of involving key stakeholders throughout the process was that vital momentum, energy, credibility and ownership of the work and recommendations was created, thereby leaving a strong base to build on in translating the recommendations into actions.

References

1. Storkey M. *London's Ethnic Minorities: one city, many communities*. London: London Research Centre, 1994.
2. London Research Centre. *Population projections of Ethnic Groups in London 1991–2011*. London: London Research Centre, 1996.
3. London Research Centre. *1995/96 Labour Force Survey – Local Authorities Database*. Cited in: Unemployed, Social Class and Occupation. *London Research Centre Bulletin* 1996; No. P74547.
4. Anderson H and Flatley J. *Contrasting London incomes: a social and spatial analysis*. London: London Research Centre, 1997.
5. National Housing Federation. *Housing for Health*. London: National Housing Federation, 1997.
6. London Research Centre. T*aking Stock of what we know: A Statistical assessment of black and minority ethnic housing needs.* London: London Research Centre, 2000.
7. Storkey M. *London's Ethnic Minorities: one city, many communities*. London: London Research Centre, 1994.
8. Home Office. *Asylum Statistics 1997*. London: Home Office, 1998.
9. Hayward A. *Tuberculosis control in London: The Need for Change. A report for the Thames Regional Directors of Public Health.* London: NHS Executive, 1998.

10. Haringey Council. *Refugees and asylum Seekers in Haringey: research project report.* London: Haringey Council, 1997.

11. Ramsay R, Gorst-Unsworth C and Turner S. Psychiatric morbidity in survivors of organised state violence including torture. A retrospective series. *British Journal of Psychiatry* 1993; 162: 55–59.

12. Brent & Harrow Health Agency, Brent & Harrow Refugee Groups, Northwest London Training and Enterprise Council. *Brent & Harrow Refugee Survey.* London: Brent & Harrow Health Agency, 1995.

13. Gammell H, Ndahiro A, Nicholas N and Windsor J. *Refugees (Political Asylum Seekers): Service Provision and Access to the NHS.* London: College of Health, 1993.

14. Carey-Wood J, Duke K, Karn V and Marshall T. *The settlement of refugees in Britain. Home Office Research Study No. 141.* London: HMSO, 1995.

15. Balarajan R. Ethnicity and variations in the nation's health. *Health Trends* 1995; 27: 114–19.

16. Nazroo J. *The Health of Britain's Ethnic Minorities: Findings from a national survey.* London: Policy Studies Institute, 1997.

17. Johnson S, Ramsay R, Thornicroft G *et al. London's Mental Health: The Report to the King's Fund London Commission.* London: King's Fund, 1997.

18. Nazroo J. *The Health of Britain's Ethnic Minorities: Findings from a national survey.* London: Policy Studies Institute, 1997.

19. Commission for Racial Equality. *The Stephen Lawrence Inquiry – Implications for Racial Equality.* London: CRE, 1999.

20. Department of Health. *The new NHS: modern, dependable. Modernising Health and Social Services.* HSC 1998/159. London: The Stationery Office, 1998.

21. NHS Executive. *Health Improvement Programmes: Planning for better health and better health care.* HSC 1998/167. Leeds: NHS Executive, 1998.

22. NHS Executive. *Health Action Zones.* Executive Letter EL(97)65. 30 October 1997.

23. NHS Executive. *Annual Planning Guidance 1999–2000.* London: The London Regional Office, London Health Strategy, May 1999.

24. Department of Health. *Health Gain for black and minority ethnic communities.* London: DoH, 1997; Department of Health. *Cumberlege Report. Department of Health Expert Maternity Working Group. Changing Childbirth.* London: HMSO, 1993.

25. Department of the Environment, Transport and the Regions. *Best Value Programme.* London: The Stationery Office, 1999.

26. Department of the Environment, Transport and the Regions. *Agenda 21 Initiative*. London: The Stationery Office, 1998.
27. NHS Executive. *The London Regional Office, London Health Strategy*. London: London Regional Office, 1999.
28. NHS Executive. *Addressing black and minority ethnic health in London – A review and recommendations*. London: NHS London Regional Office, 1999.
29. Aldous J, Bardsley M, Daniell R, Gair R, Jacobson B, Lowdell C, Morgan D, Storkey M and Taylor G. *Refugee Health in London*. London: The Health of Londoners Project, 1999; Association of London Government. *Sick of Being Excluded*. London: ALG, 2000.
30. NHS Executive. *The London Regional Office, London Health Strategy*. London, 1999.
31. White D, Phillips K and Minns A. *Women from Ethnic Minority Communities: Their Knowledge of and Needs for Health Advocacy Services in East London*. Stoke-on-Trent: Staffordshire University Press, 1999.
32. For example, see Levenson R and Gillam S. *Linkworkers in Primary Care*. London: King's Fund, 1998; and the review undertaken in Aldous J, Bardsley M, Daniell R, Gair R, Jacobson B, Lowdell C, Morgan D, Storkey M and Taylor G. *Refugee Health in London*. London: The Health of Londoners Project, 1999.
33. Fulop N and Jewkes R. Background Information. *Health Service Journal* 1992; 28–29.
34. White D, Phillips K and Minns A. *Women from Ethnic Minority Communities: Their Knowledge of and Needs for Health Advocacy Services in East London*. Stoke-on-Trent: Staffordshire University Press, 1999.
35. Mocroft I, Pharoah C and Romney-Alexander D. *Healthy Relationships: a Survey of London health authorities' and trusts' support to the voluntary sector*. Kent: Charities Aid Foundation, 1999.
36. For example, see Kapasi R and Silvera M. *The needs of Black and minority ethnic carers living in Southwark*. London: CUWG, 1998; Grant C and Deane J. *Stating the obvious – factors that influence the uptake and provision of primary care services to refugees*. London: Brixton Challenge, Lambeth, Southwark and Lewisham Health Authority, 1995; Cole M and Cheeseman C. *Opening the door: a study into the needs of people from ethnic communities with visual impairment living in the Royal Borough of Kensington and Chelsea*. Surrey: seeAbility (Association of Blind Asians), 1998.
37. Brent CHC. Voices of Women in Brent, Talking about Maternity Services. 1999.
38. Cole A. Double Jeopardy. *Health Visitor* 1996; 69(4): 131–32.
39. Islington Zairian Refugees Group. *Islington Zairian Refugees Survey Report*. London: Healthy Islington, 2000.

40. Lambeth, Southwark and Lewisham Health Authority. *Lambeth, Southwark and Lewisham Refugee Outreach Team – Annual report 1997/98*. London: Lambeth, Southwark and Lewisham Health Authority, 1998.

41. Bariso EU. *The Horn of Africa Health Research Project: An assessment of the accessibility and appropriateness of health care services to Horn of Africa (Eritrean, Ethiopian, Oromo & Somali) communities in Camden & Islington*. London: Healthy Islington and Camden & Islington Health Authority, 1997.

42. Deane J. Refugee access to primary care services. *Share* 1997; 16: 7–8.

43. Haringey Council. *Refugees and Asylum Seekers in Haringey: Research project report*. London: Haringey Council, 1997.

44. London Borough of Lewisham. *Addressing the needs of HIV and asylum seekers*. London: London Borough of Lewisham Social Services Conference, March 1999.

45. Gammell H, Ndahiro A, Nicholas N and Windsor J. *Refugees (Political Asylum Seekers): Service Provision and Access to the NHS*. London: College of Health, 1993.

2. Questionnaire analysis

This section presents the key findings of the questionnaire mapping exercise. Questionnaires were targeted at three distinct types of respondents – *those who provide health advocacy services*, *those who fund health advocacy services* and *those who provide advocacy training.*

A comprehensive mailing list was devised to cover all health and social care providers, commissioners and training agencies in London, as well as umbrella and 'link' agencies that would have knowledge of local organisations. Appendix 3 gives a detailed breakdown of agencies that we mailed and the response rate. At the beginning of the exercise we were working in the dark as only three agencies in London identified local health advocacy groups that they were aware of. In many boroughs we undertook very large mailings to ensure as wide a coverage as possible, with no knowledge of what response rate to expect. Over a six-month period, all agencies were mailed twice to maximise the response rate. We believe that the actual numbers of agencies that responded reflect a cross-section of the work that is carried out within black and minority ethnic communities with a particular focus on health advocacy support. The response rate from statutory agencies, as funders, was poorer than expected. In addition to the steps mentioned above, health authorities were specifically targeted in an attempt to get a better response as it became clear from our initial analysis that some of the health authorities that had not responded were funding a number of agencies that returned the provider questionnaire. It was less easy to pursue NHS trusts due to sheer volume and time constraints. However, it is likely that NHS trusts are not major funders of health advocacy projects, except in a small number of cases where schemes were provided within a trust.

This section is broken down into three parts:

Part 2.1, Advocacy providers in London, gives an overview of advocacy providers in the capital, the type of organisations providing this service, the type of service they provide, when and how they monitor and measure the effectiveness of their work, and which boroughs, care groups and minority ethnic groups they work with.

Part 2.2, Funding, describes the levels of funding received by groups and the level of support and funding provided by funding organisations.

Part 2.3, Training, provides an overview of training agencies, the type of courses they run, whether the courses lead to accreditation and the type of funding they receive.

In this section, we have identified agencies that provide health advocacy as their main activity as '*advocacy providers*' and those that provide some health advocacy as part of a broader pattern of services as '*generic providers*'. The distinction was made by agencies themselves and is self-explanatory. Generic providers were asked to state how much of their work comprised health advocacy. We feel this is an important comparison for this exercise as it helps to understand better the type and volume of advocacy work happening across London, which may be 'part and parcel' of everyday work for many community groups.

2.1 Advocacy providers in London

Who provides health advocacy services?

One-hundred-and-sixty-three organisations across London responded to the questionnaire for *providers of advocacy services.* Many of these organisations provide services across more than one London borough (see 'Open to the public' below). Of the 163 providers:

- 47 (29 per cent) indicated that they provided advocacy as their *main activity* ('advocacy providers')
- 116 (71 per cent) indicated that health advocacy was provided as *part of a wider range of activities* ('generic providers').

Of the 116 agencies for whom health advocacy was not their main role, over a third (38 per cent) stated that advocacy constituted 30–50 per cent of their activities. This represents a substantial amount of time dedicated to providing clients with advocacy support within this group of providers, showing that generic providers are by no means 'marginal providers'.

Table 2.1: Proportion of health advocacy work by non-main advocacy providers

Percentage proportion of health advocacy work	*Number of agencies*
10–20%	47 agencies (40%)
20–30%	25 agencies (22%)
30–50%	44 agencies (38%)

Out of all providers, a total of *52 per cent* were black and minority ethnic/refugee community groups. The majority of these were generic providers (57 per cent).

Appendix 5 shows a map of Greater London, plotting the geographical distribution of agencies that took part in the survey.

Types of services provided

To assist respondents, the questionnaire included a description of the types of activities covered by 'health advocacy' (Appendix 6 shows the provider questionnaire).

Although the majority of the agencies that indicated advocacy was their main role selected almost all the options offered on the questionnaire, as shown in Table 2.2, the predominant activities for advocacy and generic providers were enabling users to access services, followed by helping people say what their problems were and obtaining their rights. The specific activity least undertaken by both advocacy and generic providers was to represent the interests of users.

Table 2.2: Types of advocacy support provided by all providers

	Say what problems are	*Obtain rights*	*Represent interests*	*Access services needed*	*Other types of advocacy*
Advocacy	89%	87%	83%	93%	30%
Generic	73%	79%	64%	84%	32%

This indicates that for black and minority ethnic and refugee communities in London, health advocacy needs are first and foremost about simply communicating needs, obtaining basic rights and accessing services, before moving to the stage of advocates representing their interests. This was more the case with generic providers, of whom only 64 per cent undertook advocacy that involved representing rights.

Similar percentages of providers in both groups selected the 'other types of advocacy work' option to describe a broader range of work relating to advocacy. These activities indicated an understanding of advocacy that was very broadly defined and included activities such as counselling, health education, needs assessment and campaigning. Appendix 7 shows a breakdown of the other types of advocacy work described.

What type of organisations are they?

Status of advocacy providers. Eighty-four per cent of advocacy providers were based in the voluntary sector; the majority of these (80 per cent) were registered charities. Only 16 per cent of advocacy providers were from the statutory sector. All of these were NHS trust providers located within NHS trusts, apart from one that was based within a primary care group.

Status of generic providers. A greater number of generic providers, 97 per cent, were based in the voluntary sector, with 58 per cent of these being registered charities and 28 per cent identifying themselves as voluntary organisations. Of the 3 per cent based within the statutory sector, all were NHS trust providers.

Table 2.3: Status of advocacy providers

	Unreg. charity	*Reg. charity*	*Company ltd by guarantee*	*Community /voluntary group*	*NHS trust*	*Self-help group*	*Voluntary organisation*	*Other*
Advocacy	9%	80%	32%	16%	16%	7%	25%	2%
Generic	10%	58%	22%	15%	3%	3%	28%	4%
All	10%	64%	33%	15%	7%	4%	21%	4%

Size of providers. Of the 163 providers, the average number of paid staff among advocacy and generic providers who identified numbers of staff was similar. The difference between advocacy providers, where the average was 4.3, and generic providers, where the average was 4.2, was not significant.

Generic providers appeared to be more reliant on 'unpaid' staff to deliver their services, as the average number of unpaid staff was 3.1, with 62 per cent of generic providers delivering their advocacy service through unpaid staff. This compared to 45 per cent of advocacy providers. However, it is important to note that the extent of reliance on either unpaid staff or staff whose main role is not advocacy and who incorporate this function into their everyday work is widespread across advocacy and generic providers: 18 per cent of advocacy providers have no paid staff to deliver advocacy services, and the figure rises to 44 per cent for generic advocacy providers. This finding is also confirmed when we examine the average number of paid and unpaid hours of advocacy (identified by respondents) (see Table 2.5), which shows that all service providers undertake more 'unpaid' hours of advocacy than paid.

Table 2.4: Size of advocacy providers

	Average number of paid advocacy workers	*Average number of unpaid advocacy workers*	*Percentage of organisations with no paid staff*	*Percentage of organisations with no unpaid staff*
Advocacy	4.3	2.1	18%	45%
Generic	4.2	3.1	44%	62%

Volume of service provided

The number of hours spent doing advocacy was completed by 59 per cent of providers. Analysis shows that:

- advocacy providers offer a slightly greater volume of advocacy services than generic providers, from their average weekly hours (paid and unpaid) spent
- amazingly, advocacy providers are not paid for two-thirds (66 per cent) of the advocacy hours they deliver. This figure is slightly less for generic providers, who are not paid for 60 per cent of the advocacy hours they deliver.

This highlights the fact that a greater proportion – or even the majority – of advocacy work in all provider organisations appears to be undertaken by volunteers.

Table 2.5: Number of hours of advocacy services provided by organisations

	Advocacy providers	*Generic providers*
Average weekly number of paid hours	14.9	14.8
Average weekly number of unpaid hours	29.23	22.0
Total number of weekly hours per organisation	44.13	36.8

Communities served by advocacy providers

Volume of work undertaken with black and minority ethnic communities. The majority of the 163 providers that responded undertook over 75 per cent or more of their work with black and minority ethnic and refugee communities. The ratios were similar among all providers, the differences being that:

- advocacy providers carried out a higher proportion of their advocacy work with black and minority ethnic groups
- all advocacy providers undertook at least 25 per cent or more of their work with black and minority ethnic communities, whereas 13 per cent of generic providers undertook less than 25 per cent.

Table 2.6: Percentage of work specifically undertaken with black and minority ethnic communities

	0–25%	*26–50%*	*51–75%*	*76–100%*
Advocacy	0	13	17	70
Generic	13	5	8	74

Table 2.7 overleaf highlights the communities that are most commonly targeted by the providers who responded. The ethnic groups shown are summarised using the main 1991 Census categories.

Black and minority ethnic communities served by advocacy providers. The groups that are targeted most frequently by providers are Black African (who receive 33 per cent of advocacy services) and Bangladeshi (31 per cent), closely followed by other ethnic groups (27 per cent), Indian, Pakistani and Black Caribbean groups. Table 2.7 also shows that once this is mapped against the distribution of black and minority ethnic communities across London as a whole, the proportion of provision does correlate for most groups except Bangladeshis, who comprise 1.65 per cent of the population but receive about 31 per cent of the targeted services. This finding is not surprising against evidence about the level of socio-economic disadvantage experienced by this group in terms of employment, long-term limiting illness and levels of overcrowding, which exceed that for other minority ethnic groups.[1]

When all providers are compared, we can see that there are more advocacy services available from generic providers to all the key ethnic groups in the main Census categories.

Table 2.7: Summary of black and minority ethnic communities served by advocacy providers

Ethnic group	*Percentage of minority ethnic groups in London population*	*Percentage of all providers*	*Percentage of advocacy providers*	*Percentage of generic providers*
All ethnic groups	24.9	11	3	8
Any other ethnic group	2.38	27	9	16
Bangladeshi	1.65	31	11	20
Black African	3.72	33	13	20
Black Caribbean	4.71	23	9	14
Black Other	1.61	5	2	3
Chinese	1.02	9	4	5
Indian	5.84	26	9	15
Pakistani	1.75	24	9	13
White	72.12	9	2	7

Source: London Research Centre 1999 totals and percentages from 1998 round.

Refugee communities served by providers. Table 2.8 shows the main refugee categories identified within the *Refugee Health in London* Survey (the most current source of refugee numbers in London as identified by the London Research Centre) mapped against the percentage of the total number of providers, advocacy providers and generic providers offering services to that group.

The pattern of provision across refugee groups shows that all providers cover a broad range of refugee groups. Although the volume of provision among advocacy providers and generic providers is difficult to quantify, more advocacy providers (75 per cent) identified that, overall, they targeted one or more refugee communities than generic providers (66 per cent). In terms of broad geographical regions, the highest overall coverage was for groups from Africa, followed by Eastern Europe and, last, the Middle East. There were a few groups with a higher coverage, which included Ethiopians (9 per cent), Ugandans (8 per cent), Sudanese (7 per cent) and Rwandans (7 per cent). Exceptional coverage overall was shown for Somali refugees, who received targeted or specific services from 27 per cent of providers, were covered by 36 per cent of advocacy providers and 20 per cent of generic providers. This may indicate that there is a greater need for advocacy among Somali communities, which has been identified and responded to, as available data indicates that Somali groups in London are not substantially larger than other groups.[††, 2]

[††] For example, Somalis comprised 8 per cent of total asylum applications made to the Home Office in 1997, just ahead of refugees from the former Yugoslavia (7 per cent) and USSR (6 per cent).

Table 2.8: Breakdown of refugee communities served by providers

Refugee communities in London	*Percentage of all providers offering a service*	*Percentage of advocacy providers*	*Percentage of generic providers*
All	14.0	14.0	15.0
Any other refugee group	22.0	29.0	19.0
Afghan	4	2	4
Albanian	5	11.0	3
Algerian	0.6	0	1
Angolan	7.5	23.0	2
Bulgarian	2	5	1
Chilean	0.6	0	1
Chinese	0.6	2	0
Colombian	1	0	2
Cypriot	2	5	0
Czech and Slovak	3	11.0	0
Ecuadorian	0.6	0	1
Ethiopian (inc. Eritrean)	9	16.0	7
Former USSR (inc. Armenian)	0	0	0
Former Yugoslavia (inc. Kosovan and Croatian)	2	2	2
Ghanaian	6	18	2
Hungarian	0	0	0
Iranian	6	9	5
Iraqi	5	5	5
Kenyan	6	18.0	2
Kurdish	6	11.0	4
Lebanese	0.5	0	3
Liberian	6	19.0	1
Libyan	0.5	2	0
Nigerian	6	18.0	2
Polish	2	5	1
Roma (Romany)	0.5	0	1
Romanian	1	5	0
Rwandan	7	23.0	1
Sierra Leonean	6	18.0	2
Sinhalese	0.5	2	0
Somali	27.0	36.0	20.0
Sudanese	7.5	23.0	2
Syrian	0	0	0
Tamil	2.5	1	3
Togolese/Ivorian	5	16	1
Turkish	3	3	2
Ugandan	8	9	2
Zairian (Democratic Republic of Congo)	6	18	2

List of refugee groups source: Aldous J, Bardsley M, Daniell R, Gair R, Jacobson B, Lowdell C, Morgan D, Storkey M and Taylor G. *Refugee Health in London.* London: The Health of Londoners Project, 1999.

Sectors covered by health advocacy providers

For all providers, primary care was where they targeted most of their health advocacy services and hence resources. Generic providers targeted more of their services than advocacy providers. This suggests that clients are expressing greater levels of need in primary care than in other areas.

Different patterns of provision emerged among providers. For advocacy providers, most of their services were spread evenly between primary care, hospitals and social services. A larger majority of generic providers provided services in primary care, followed by social services, the voluntary sector and various local authority departments. Local authority departments mentioned most were housing, followed by education, police and benefits. The types of voluntary sector advocacy services that providers mentioned were community health promotion, advice, counselling, referrals, interpreting, support groups, information and training.

Table 2.9: Sectors covered by providers

	Primary care	*Hospitals*	*Social services*	*Other local authority*	*Voluntary sector*
Advocacy	67%	65%	65%	39%	19%
Generic	80%	66%	70%	49%	50%

A significant finding within this breakdown is the high level of service provision in primary care, compared to the low level of identified investment. This may be because health authorities still hold the majority of funding for work in this sector, and many health authorities did not identify separately their primary care funding. There were also few primary care trusts in London at the time of the research. However, as primary care trusts establish themselves and take greater control of identifying local needs and developing local services, investment should be expected to increase, as the primary care sector is targeted by the greatest numbers of both advocacy and generic providers.

Figure 2.1: Percentage of sectors covered by advocacy providers (n=47)

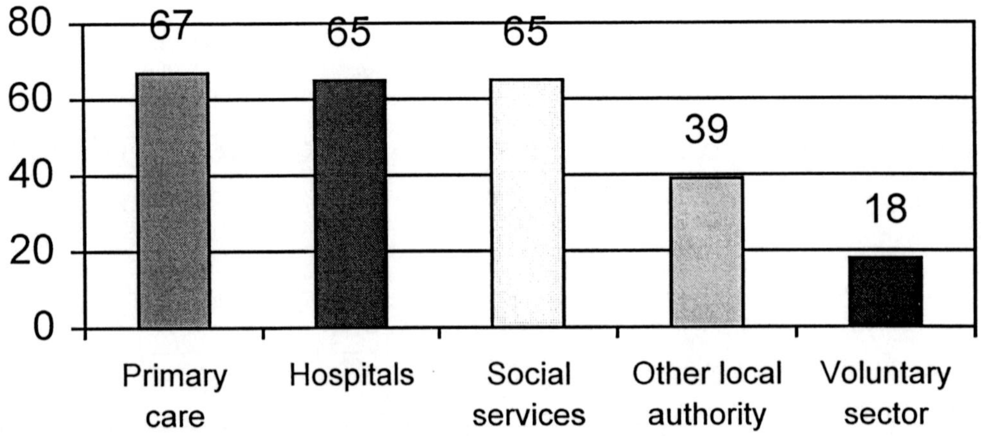

Figure 2.2: Percentage of sectors covered by generic providers (n=116)

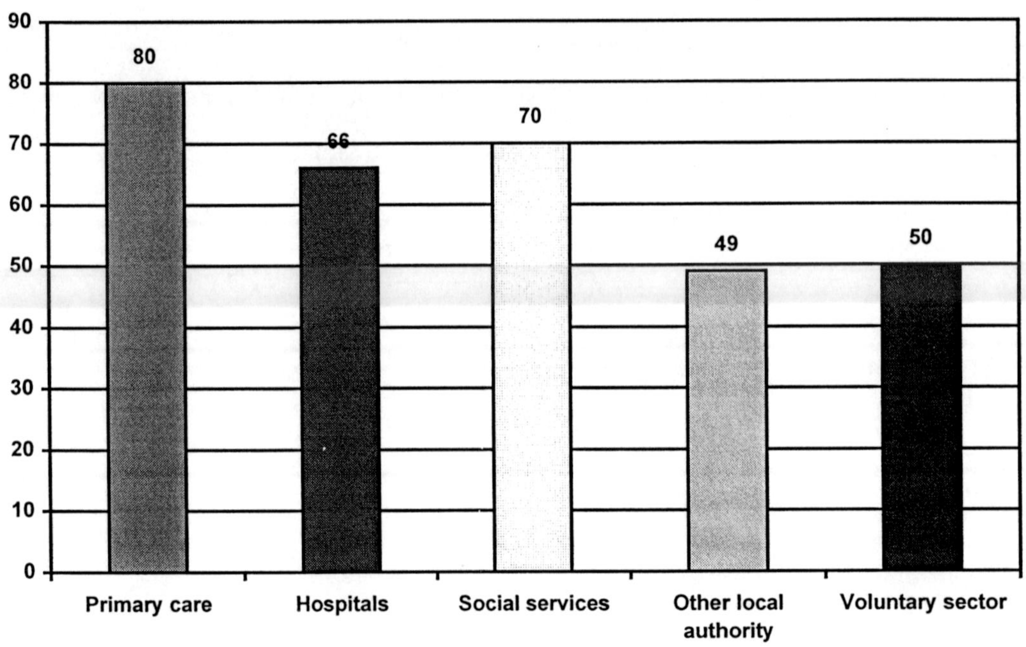

Care groups covered

For all providers, the highest proportion of their services went to older people, young people, people with mental health needs and children and families. This matches the high levels of needs of older, more settled minority ethnic communities, the over-representation of mental health-related problems among minority ethnic communities and the fact that London receives about 85 per cent of the refugees and asylum seekers settling in the UK, who tend to fall into the younger age range. The high proportion of services provided to older people reiterates the continuing needs of black elders, which are likely to grow as the average age of black and minority ethnic populations increases in London.

There were no marked differences in the pattern of coverage among providers. Advocacy providers offered more services to 'young people', children and families and people with mental health needs. This probably reflects the slightly higher number (75 per cent) of advocacy providers that work with refugee communities compared to generic providers.

The lowest care group coverage was for people with physical disabilities and learning difficulties, highlighting a potential gap in service provision for these care groups that needs to be addressed.

Figure 2.3: Percentage of care groups covered by advocacy provid ers (n=47)

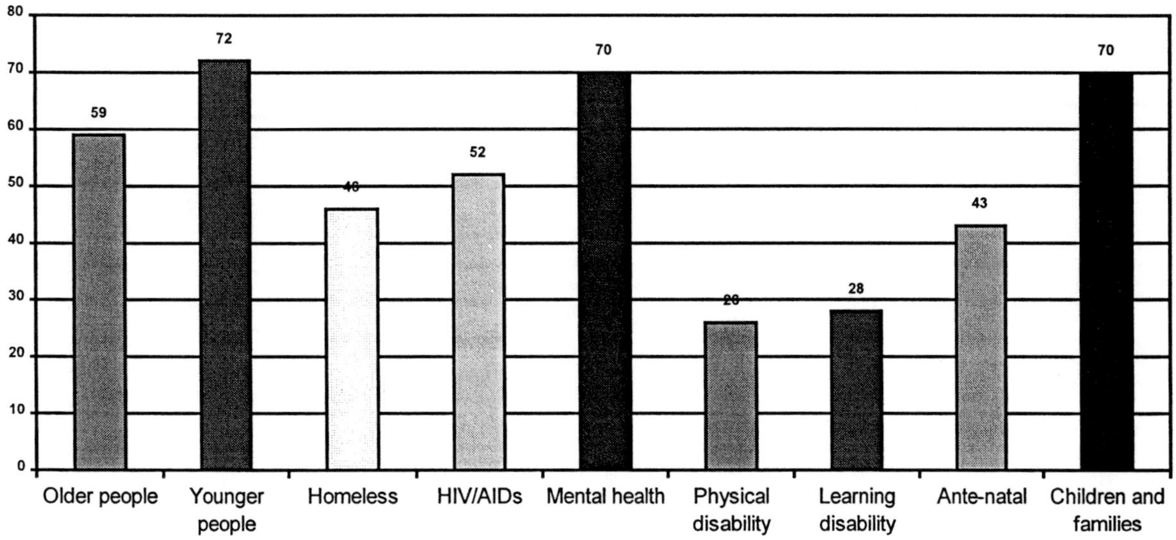

Figure 2.4: Percentage of care groups served by generic providers (n=116)

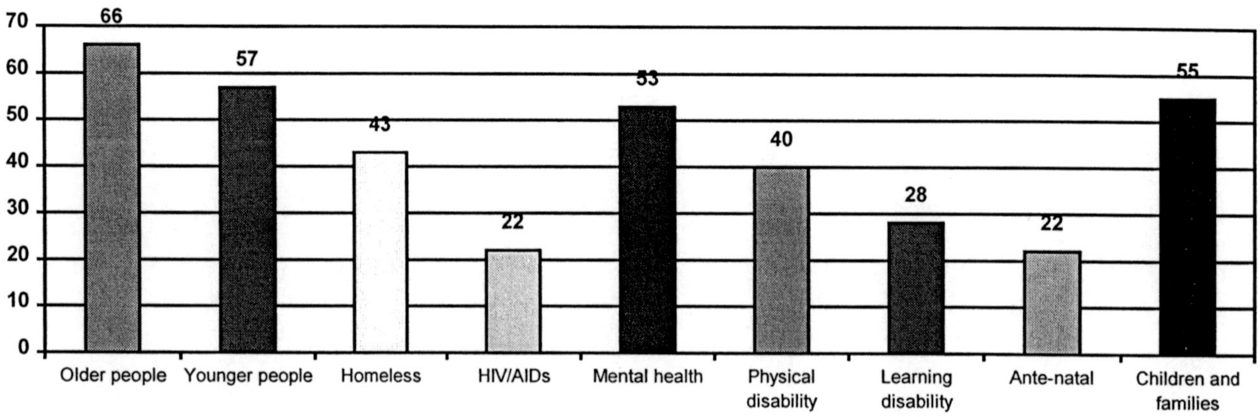

Catchment areas

Table 2.10: Catchment areas of all providers

	One borough	*More than one borough*	*HA area*	*Specific trusts*	*GP practice*	*Other catchment*
Advocacy	13	32	4	3	0	0
Generic	37	78	13	3	1	9

The majority of agencies operated on a borough-wide basis with very few working in smaller catchment areas. Two out of the three providers who worked for specific NHS trusts stated that they worked for mental health trusts. The majority of agencies working on a borough-wide basis operated in more than one borough, often as a result of meeting specific needs of particular minority ethnic communities. For this reason, a number of groups stated that they worked across London.

The distribution of providers by borough has been compared to the most recent figures of boroughs with:

- the highest concentrations of minority ethnic populations[3]
- the highest percentage of asylum seekers[4]
- the highest percentage of asylum-seeking households in temporary accommodation[5]
- significant numbers of refugee children (Refugee Council estimates).[6]

In relation to these comparisons, the findings show that boroughs with high concentrations of black and minority ethnic communities and refugees and asylum seekers do have a higher number of advocacy and generic providers. Thus, Barnet, for example, has the highest number of overall health advocacy providers, because even though Barnet has a lower overall minority ethnic population than a number of other boroughs, it has one of the highest percentages of asylum seekers settling in the area.

The two boroughs in which one would have expected a higher number of advocacy providers are Hackney and Ealing. Hackney has seven providers and is the borough with the highest percentage of refugee children. It has one of the highest percentages of overall black and minority ethnic communities and a high percentage of asylum-seeking households in temporary accommodation. Ealing has an equally high overall minority ethnic population and one of the highest percentages of settling asylum seekers and asylum-seeking households in temporary accommodation. Ealing has a total of eight providers, six of which are generic.

The boroughs with the highest number of advocacy providers were Newham (11), Camden (eight), Islington (eight) and Lewisham (seven). This highlights the fact that the needs of minority ethnic populations are being addressed in these boroughs with the statutory sector supporting the development of advocacy providers. Newham, for example, is the borough with the second highest minority ethnic population in London and the second highest numbers of refugee children.

The highest numbers of generic providers were in Westminster and Redbridge. This shows that communities in these areas have organised themselves to meet needs and, possibly, gaps in statutory sector provision to meet these needs. Westminster, for example, has the highest number of refugee families in temporary accommodation and a high percentage of settling asylum seekers.

Table 2.11: Distribution of providers by borough

Borough	*Number of advocacy providers*	*Number of generic providers*	*Total number of providers*
Barnet	7	9	16
Brent	8	6	14
Camden	8	6	14
Lewisham	7	7	14
Newham	11	3	14
Tower Hamlets	6	7	13
Lambeth	5	7	12
Islington	8	3	11
Southwark	4	7	11
Haringey	4	6	10
Merton	4	6	10
Redbridge	2	8	10
Westminster	2	8	10
Kensington & Chelsea	3	6	9
Richmond	3	6	9
Ealing	2	6	8
Enfield	3	5	8
Hammersmith & Fulham	3	5	8
Bromley	5	3	8
Hackney	5	2	7
City	4	2	6
Greenwich	3	3	6
Harrow	4	2	6
Hillingdon	2	4	6
Kingston	4	2	6
Sutton	2	4	6
Wandsworth	5	1	6
Croydon	1	4	5
Havering	2	3	5
Waltham Forest	1	4	5
Hounslow	2	2	4

Table 2.12: Boroughs with the highest numbers of black and minority ethnic communities and refugees and asylum seekers

Borough	*Approx.percentage of BMEC (Based on 1991 Census projections – likely to be underestimated)*	*Percentage of asylum seekers (Based on ONS population estimates)*	*Percentage of asylum-seeking households in temporary accommodation (to Sept. 1998)*	*Percentage of refugee children in London boroughs (Based On Refugee Council estimates, 1997)*
Brent	45	6.1	4.1	7.3
Newham	43	3.8	3.4	9.5
Tower Hamlets	36	2.8	3.4	2.4
Hackney	34	4.1	5.8	10.2
Ealing	33	6.3	7.1	5.9
Lambeth	31	4.2	4.4	0.4
Haringey	30	4.7	5.3	6.5
Harrow	27	2.9	2.3	1.8
Waltham Forest	26	2.2	2.1	2.3
Hounslow	25	3.0	1.9	2.8
Southwark	25	3.2	2.6	3.3
Lewisham	22	2.2	2.0	5.4
Westminster	22	6.5	11.4	3.1
Wandsworth	21	3.9	1.8	1.8
Barnet	19	6.5	3.2	5.4

Open to the public

Five advocacy providers offered their services for less than 35 hours per week. The majority of main advocacy providers who identified numbers of hours of availability were available for 35 hours or more, with one being available for 80 hours per week. All these providers offered their services during office hours, with 14 per cent being available at weekends and in the evenings.

Eleven generic providers offered their services for less than 35 hours per week. The majority provided their services for between 20 and 35 hours per week. Generic providers were slightly more accessible to the public out of office hours than main providers, with 16 per cent providing a service in the evening and 20 per cent being available at weekends.

Table 2.13: Hours available to clients by providers

	Totals	*Available office hours*	*Available weekends*	*Available evenings*
Advocacy	47	100%	14%	14%
Generic	116	79%	16%	20%

Main methods of referral

Analysis of the main methods of referral shows quite different patterns between providers. For advocacy providers, the majority of referrals are from the statutory sector (45 per cent), followed by self-referral (36 per cent). A total of 20 per cent of their referrals come from the voluntary sector and through other methods. Other methods of referral identified by advocacy providers were outreach into the community, friends, word of mouth and via the Internet.

For generic providers, almost three-quarters of referrals (72 per cent) are by self-referral, with 13 per cent from the statutory sector, 10 per cent through other methods and 5 per cent from the voluntary sector. The other methods of referral described were referrals from other users, friends and family and community members, through word of mouth networks, visiting hostels and outreach work.

These differences indicate that statutory sector agencies are more likely to refer to main advocacy providers. This may simply be because they may be more aware of them or have greater confidence in their abilities to provide advocacy services. Direct knowledge of generic providers appears to be far greater among service users. Service users may also find it easier to access or approach generic providers directly, as they may be able to identify more people offering the service (because more generic providers are black and minority ethnic and refugee community-based organisations) or a greater provision of languages available. The questionnaire for providers did not ask for information about which language services were available, which would have been a useful comparison.

Table 2.14: Main methods of referrals received by providers (shown as percentages of the total methods identified by providers)

	Self-referrals	*Referrals from the statutory sector*	*Referrals from the voluntary sector*	*Other methods of referral*
Advocacy	36%	45%	14%	6%
Generic	72%	13%	5%	10%

What difference does advocacy make?

How do projects know if their service is being effective? The most frequent method of measuring and assessing the effectiveness of advocacy services used by all providers was informal user feedback, followed by recording the number of clients seen. Marginally more advocacy providers monitor complaints and feedback from referral agencies and health professionals, but all providers used the other methods equally (see Table 2.15).

Analysis of descriptions of the methods used by providers reveals that advocacy providers do not use more developed methods of measuring effectiveness than generic providers. However, advocacy providers do use measures such as monitoring of complaints, referral agency and health professional feedback, user surveys and numbers of clients seen to a greater extent than generic providers. This indicates that more advocacy providers have, for example, more developed internal mechanisms (such as complaints systems).

In total, very few providers monitored the outcomes of their advocacy work. However, more generic providers (6 per cent) stated that they used outcome measurements such as user evaluation of outcome achievement, results achieved through advocacy intervention, user ability to access services and outcomes of contact than advocacy providers (2 per cent). It is certainly the case that generic providers have less stable and more short-term sources of funding and this may have been an initial catalyst for some providers to develop more 'rigorous' methods to monitor and evaluate their service to justify the continuation of their funding. Appendix 8 identifies the methods that all providers described for measuring and assessing the effectiveness of their services.

It is therefore clear that monitoring effectiveness is a largely 'undeveloped' area in the field of advocacy.

Table 2.15: How effectiveness is measured by providers

	Informal user feedback	*User surveys*	*Complaints*	*Referral agencies' feedback*	*Health professionals' feedback*	*Number of clients seen*	*Other measures*
Advocacy	86%	59%	70%	70%	66%	84%	16%
Generic	73%	54%	54%	44%	52%	57%	19%

Links with key agencies

Overall, providers reported that their best links were with health authorities (62 per cent), closely followed by social services (61 per cent), then local councils for voluntary services (51 per cent). A majority of providers indicated that they had no links with, and in many cases had not heard of, Health Action Zones (85 per cent), Healthy Living Centres (91 per cent), New Deal (92 per cent) and urban regeneration (84 per cent).[‡‡] This finding may in part be explained by the fact that there are only four Health Action Zones in London and not all areas have Health Living Centres or are involved in urban regeneration programmes. This noted, the figures are still high and could indicate that, at local levels, mainstream statutory agencies are either unaware of agencies providing advocacy or do not consult and involve them in local initiatives.

The most striking differences to emerge when links between providers are compared are:

- advocacy providers reported noticeably better links with NHS trusts, local networks, community forums, the Community Health Council (CHC) and local councils for voluntary services. For example, at least half or more generic providers reported poor or no links with the CHC, community forums and local networks
- advocacy providers reported marginally worse links than generic providers with Racial Equality Councils, with 45 per cent of advocacy providers having no links with or not having heard of Racial Equality Councils compared to 40 per cent of generic providers
- advocacy providers reported the worst links with GP practices and primary care groups. Even though generic providers reported better links, 37 per cent still reported no links with GP practices and 39 per cent no links with primary care groups.

From this analysis, it is clear that a number of 'mainstream' umbrella groups such as Community Health Councils, councils for voluntary services and local networks and forums that may be set up to embrace, support and pass information onto advocacy providers are not reaching and involving generic providers.

---

‡‡ See Appendix 9 for a more detailed breakdown of links.

2.2 Funding

How are health advocacy services funded?

A total of 115 agencies (71 per cent of the sample) indicated that they received some form of funding for the services they provided. The proportion of funded providers was higher among advocacy providers (84 per cent) than generic providers (67 per cent).

The significance of these findings is that 16 per cent of advocacy providers do not receive any funding and a third (33 per cent) of generic providers in London are also carrying out advocacy work for which they are not being funded.

The majority of providers who identified the length of their funding were also funded on a short-term (less than a one- or two-year) basis. Over a third of advocacy providers (37 per cent) are funded for less than two years. However, more advocacy providers (16 per cent) are funded on a longer-term (more than five-year) basis, compared to generic providers, of whom only 6 per cent were funded for longer than five years.

Table 2.16: Funded or not?

	Funded	*Not funded*	*Funded for less than 2 years*	*Funded for longer than 5 years*
All providers	71%	29%	-	-
Advocacy providers	84%	16%	37%	16%
Generic providers	67%	33%	20%	6%

Funding sources

Table 2.17 below shows where providers receive their funding from, and the total amount. Table 2.18 shows the overall percentage of providers who receive funding from a particular source. The total identified funding received by advocacy providers is approximately £2.6 million. The total identified funding received by generic providers is approximately £2.1

million. *For the purposes of comparison*[§§] *only, this shows approximately £161,908 per agency per annum for advocacy providers and approximately £25,056 for generic providers!*

When these annual funding figures are compared to the volume of service provided, calculated by dividing the total number of hours spent per year by each group undertaking advocacy work (including the number of unpaid hours) over the amount of funding received for advocacy, it reveals that advocacy providers also receive more funding for the actual advocacy hours they provide. These comparative figures need to be treated with caution as we have used simple methods of calculation that do not take into account other running costs, capital overheads, etc., and are based on volume of service provided based on numbers of hours stated by providers (as volume of client contact was not collected). However, the figures highlight an important difference in the pattern of funding across the two groups, that is advocacy providers receive more funding to undertake advocacy work than generic providers.

The funding patterns for providers have some similarities and some key differences:

- health authorities are the largest funders indicated *by all providers*, providing more funding to more providers
- *advocacy providers* are more successful in securing larger amounts of funding for health advocacy work from health authorities, trusts and PCGs
- *generic providers* are more successful in securing funds to undertake health advocacy work from social services, joint finance, local and central Government sources
- *generic providers* have a broader range of funding sources, from which they acquire smaller amounts of funding.

Table 2.17: Funding sources and amounts

	HA	*Joint Finance*	*NHS trust*	*PCG*	*SSD*	*Local gov.*	*Central Gov.*	*Charitable trust*	*National Lottery*	*Fund-raising events*	*Public appeal*	*Mem-bers*	*Private donations*	*Other funding*	*Total*
Advocacy	£1,154,297	£120,000	£471,905	£10,000	£61,000	£85,436	£30,000	£258,500	£133,463	£4000	£0	£0	£0	£323,000	£2,651,601
	(20)	(10)	(10)	(1)	(8)	(6)	(2)	(6)	(6)	(1)				(3)	
Generic	£641,996	£182,360	£153,532	£0	£203,650	£199,750	£56,000	£358,333	£318,163	£4150	£200	£1620	£8050	£5465	£2,133,269
	(21)	(12)	(6)		(12)	(8)	(2)	(21)	(14)	(4)	(1)	(3)	(4)	(2)	

Note: The number of providers who receive funding from that funding source is shown in brackets.

[§§] Averages calculated take into account organisations that did not identify funding.

Table 2.18: Where providers get their funding from

	HA	Joint Finance	NHS trust	PCG	SSD	Local gov.	Central Gov.	Charitable trust	National Lottery	Fund-raising events	Public appeal	Members	Private donations	Other funding
Advocacy	45%	2%	23%	2%	18%	14%	4.5%	14%	14%	2%	-	-	-	6%
Generic	18%	10%	5%	-	10%	7%	2%	14.5%	12%	4%	1%	3%	4%	2%

Funding analysis for specific minority ethnic groups

The analysis of funding allocated for advocacy work being undertaken for specific minority ethnic groups shows that:

- all the main ethnic groups broken down by the Census categories receive some funding to undertake advocacy work
- the worst-funded minority ethnic target group of users are those in the 'Black Other' category. Only 50 per cent of their advocacy work is funded, although we are unable to identify which precise groups these were as providers did not identify them. The next least well-funded were organisations targeting all ethnic groups – 35 per cent of their advocacy work was not funded – closely followed by those targeting Pakistani groups, 33 per cent of whose work was not funded
- the most successful groups in receiving funding to undertake health advocacy work were Chinese and white communities, who have 93 per cent and 86 per cent of their advocacy work funded, respectively.

Table 2.19: Funding analysis for services provided for specific minority ethnic groups

Ethnic group	*Number of all providers offering specific or targeted services*	*Percentage of funded providers*	*Percentage of unfunded providers*
All ethnic groups	17 (11%)	65%	35%
Any other ethnic group	43 (27%)	74%	26%
Bangladeshi	50 (31%)	70%	30%
Black African	53 (33%)	70%	30%
Black Caribbean	36 (23%)	75%	25%
Black Other	8 (5%)	50%	50%
Chinese	15 (9%)	93%	7%
Indian	41 (26%)	73%	27%
Pakistani	39 (24%)	67%	33%
White	14 (9%)	86%	14%

Appendix 10 shows the funding allocated for advocacy work with specific refugee communities and reveals that 35 per cent of work that organisations are undertaking with all refugee communities is unfunded. The breakdown by individual refugee group shows that:

- most advocacy work with the majority of refugee groups identified in London receives some form of funding
- groups undertaking advocacy work that currently receive no funding are groups targeting Chilean, Columbian, Ecuadorian, Lebanese and Roma (or Romany) communities
- other groups who have at least 25 per cent or more of advocacy work not funded are groups targeting Afghan (67 per cent unfunded), Bulgarian (37 per cent unfunded), Ethiopian (27 per cent unfunded), Iranian (50 per cent unfunded), Iraqi (50 per cent unfunded), Kurdish (30 per cent unfunded) and Somali (26 per cent unfunded) communities.

Funders' response to black and minority ethnic initiatives

A total of 18 funding agencies responded to the questionnaire for funding agencies (see Table 2.21 for a detailed list). This response was lower than expected for some funding bodies, such as local and health authorities, when compared to the number of providers across London that identified certain funding bodies as their funders.

Table 2.20: Comparison of funding body responses with number of times identified as source of funding

Type of funding agency	*Response to questionnaire*	*Mentioned as funding source by advocacy providers*
Health authority	5	41
NHS trust	4	16
Joint Finance	1	13
PCG	0	1
SSD	0	20
Local government	1	14
Central Government	1 (Home Office)	4
Charitable trust	7	27
National Lottery	0	20

Of the funding agencies that responded, seven stated that they had specific policies or existing policies that took special account of funding black and minority ethnic organisations. Of those that had such policies, six had funded black and minority ethnic schemes in the last five years and four that had not mentioned having a specific policy had funded schemes in the same period.

The total investment in black and minority ethnic projects indicated from funders who responded is £6.8 million (£6,863,163) over a one-year period to the end of March 2000. Projected investment identified by funders to April 2001 is just over £6 million (£6,492,897) for a one-year period. This indicates that, from the funders who have responded, *overall investment in this area will decrease* slightly. While not all investment was made directly in black and minority ethnic organisations, a large proportion of the future funding was earmarked by funders for services to black and minority ethnic communities.

Table 2.21: Funding agency contributions to health advocacy

Organisation	*Funding provided over last financial year to 31 March 2000*	*Funding available from 1 April 2000*	*Likely to invest in the future?*	*Policy to fund black and minority ethnic groups*
ACU – Home Office	£0	£0	Yes	No
Baring Foundation	£7270	£0	No	No
Barking and Havering Health Authority	£252,000	£292,000	Yes	Yes
Barnet Health Authority	£88,017	£108,000	No	No
Bridge House Estates Trust Fund	£75,000	Ongoing roll-over of funding indicated	Yes	Yes
Carnegie Trust UK	£0	£0	No	No
Comic Relief	£0	£0	Yes	Yes, as part of refugee programme
Consortium on Opportunities for Volunteering	£229,000	£2,000,000	Yes	Yes, as part of black and minority ethnic programme
East London and City Health Authority	£2,494,420	£2,473,753	No	Yes
Enfield and Haringey Health Authority	£268,000	£300,000	Yes	Yes
Great Ormond Street Hospital	Funding provided for one worker, amount unspecified	Funding available for one worker, amount unspecified	Yes	No
KCW HA & Joint Finance	£2,451,045	Approx. £1 million	Yes	Yes – levels of need and gaps for refugees and asylum seekers monitored
King's Fund	£195,984	£1,000,000*	Yes	Yes
Kingston Hospitals NHS Trust	£0	£0	No	No
London Borough of Camden	£120,900	£120,000	Yes	Yes
London Borough Grants	£68,263 (for specific minority ethnic health initiatives) £406,120 (for generic advocacy schemes)	Funding available, precise amount unspecified	Yes	Yes
Mary Kincross Charitable Trust	£0	£0	No	No
Newham Healthcare NHS Trust	£199,144	£199,144	Yes	No
Riverside Community Health Care NHS Trust	£8000	Funding available, amount unspecified	Yes	No
Totals	£6,863,163	£6,492,897		

**This figure will be spent on strategic development of services rather than actual provision of advocacy services and so has not been included in the total figures of future funding available.*

It is difficult to draw any conclusions from the data presented here regarding the appropriateness of the level of investment indicated related to the need for investment in advocacy services to black and minority ethnic communities. Equally, comparison would have to be made against the overall level of investment in such work within the voluntary sector as a whole (which is where the vast majority of these agencies are located), for which we have not collected data. What does emerge from the analysis, though, is:

- a sizeable majority of organisations undertaking advocacy work are not funded to provide this service (16 per cent for advocacy providers and 33 per cent for generic providers)
- of those that are funded, in spite of similar levels of service provision, advocacy providers are better resourced
- the majority of advocacy hours provided by main advocacy and generic providers are not paid for
- there are no marked differences in funding for providers targeting the main minority ethnic groups from the Census categories
- advocacy providers targeting work with refugee communities are less well-funded, with some refugee groupings receiving no funding and a number of others indicating a higher proportion of no funding
- the overall level of investment in this area of work by funders who responded will decrease slightly over the 2000/2001 financial year.

In general terms, recent research into the level of spending across London in the voluntary sector by major funders points to lower than average levels of spending within black and minority ethnic communities compared to their make-up of the population. The research points to about 2.9 per cent of health spending in the voluntary sector going to black and minority ethnic agencies.[7] The sourcing and availability of funding for their advocacy services was a key area of concern identified by the majority of agencies that responded to the mapping (see Section 3).

Non-financial support provided by funding agencies

The most commonly identified areas where funding agencies provided non-financial support were in offering their own staff to assist projects working on specific issues, in supporting the infrastructure development of organisations and in providing external consultancy support. This focus reflected awareness by these funding agencies of some of the key organisational development concerns that smaller agencies, in particular, have to address.

Table 2.22: Number of funding agencies providing non-financial support to funded projects

Management training	*Consultancy support*	*Own staff on specific issues*	*Opportunities to network*	*Infrastructure development*	*Other support*
2	5	8	3	7	1

2.3 Training

How are advocates trained?

Ninety-three (58 per cent of the sample) of all the agencies that responded indicated that they required the advocates who worked for them to receive some form of training. Fifty-six agencies (35 per cent) indicated that they provided training internally and 56 (35 per cent) used external trainers. Thirty-eight agencies mentioned that the training their advocates received led to some sort of qualification and, of these, 16 were accredited qualifications. Table 2.23 below summarises the key differences between advocacy and generic providers.

Table 2.23: Summary of training received by advocates from providers

	Require min. Qualifications	*Advocates receive training*	*Training leads to qualification*	*Training leads to accreditation*	*Training provided internally*	*Training provided externally*
Advocacy	36%	80%	38%	15%	47%	58%
Generic	43%	49%	18%	8%	30%	34%
All	47%	58%	24%	14%	35%	40%

The key differences between providers in the training that their advocates receive were:

- more advocates working for advocacy providers receive some form of training
- more generic providers require their advocates to have some form of minimum qualification
- more of the training received by advocates working for advocacy providers leads to qualifications and accreditation.

Who provides training?

Eight agencies responded to the questionnaire for training providers. Trainers described ten different courses on advocacy or work related to advocacy. Six of the courses specifically targeted black and minority ethnic communities.

How is training funded?

With the exception of two training providers, all the courses were funded from a designated budget and did not require participants to pay. Only one training agency had access to secure mainstream funding; all other agencies had developed their courses with 'one-off' grants and had to re-apply annually for funds.

Many of the training agencies highlighted the fact that the focus of their courses was determined by the criteria attached to funding. For example, one agency was unable to use the term 'advocacy' in the title of the training because the European funding that they received did not recognise the term 'advocacy' and instead used 'mediation'.

What type of accreditation models exist?

Providers used two types of accreditation:

- accreditation of courses to levels 2 and 3 by the London Open College Network
- accreditation to NVQ level.

What type of training exists for bi-lingual advocates?

There are currently no combined training courses for bi-lingual advocates. The Urban Learning Foundation offers a community interpreting module as a separate unit to the advocacy module and a number of further education colleges offer interpreting modules and courses, which advocates would need to undertake separately from specific advocacy training. Thus, individuals who are employed as bi-lingual advocates and who have not received formal interpreting training are reliant on employers to ensure that they receive both types of training.

Table 2.24: Profile of training providers

Organisation	*Training type*	*Specific to BMEC?*	*When available?*	*Funded through participants?*	*Funded by other sources*	*Plan to run again?*
Barnet General Hospital	Health promotion workshops	No	One per month	No	Yes	Yes
UK Coalition of People Living with HIV/AIDS	Everything you wanted to know about advocacy but were afraid to ask: basic introductions to concepts and issues	Yes	By arrangement	No	Yes	Yes
Making Training Work	LOCN accredited Advocacy and Mediation in Health	Yes	As and when required by potential employees and organisations	No	Yes	Yes
Urban Learning Foundation	LOCN units: Advocacy and Mediation in Health	Yes	Negotiated on demand	Yes	Yes	Yes
Croydon CETS	Advocacy in Health – LOCN accredited	Yes	Once a year	No	Yes	Yes
SRB Advocacy Project	Advocacy skills core competence training	No	February 2000	No	Yes	Yes
Westminster Advocacy Services for Senior Residents	3-day training for volunteers	Yes		No	No	No
Citizen Advocacy Information and Training	Mental health difficulties and older people	No	30 May 2000	Yes	Yes	Yes

Table 2.25: Advocacy training courses

Organisation	*Project provided for*	*Course title(s)*
Barnet General Hospital	Linkworkers and professionals	Health Promotion Workshops
UK Coalition of People Living with HIV/AIDS	African community groups	• Advocacy – all you needed to know • Participation in joint commissions team • Peer group advocacy • Working alongside people with HIV infection
Making Training Work	Manor Garden Health Advocacy Project	Making Training Work
Urban Learning Foundation	Advocates and linkworkers in the public or voluntary sector in ELCHA area	Advocacy and Mediation in Health
Croydon CETS	An advent education organisation for minority ethnic groups	Advocacy and Mediation Health
SRB Advocacy Project	People in Newham working as or wanting to be advocates	Advocacy Skills Core Competence training
Westminster Advocacy Services for Senior Residents	Our own volunteers targets representing all communities in London	Advocacy and Older People
Citizen Advocacy Information and Training	Staff and managers of citizen advocacy schemes. Advocates and service providers and officers with an interest in CA	Mental Health Difficulties and Older People

References

1. For example, see figures cited in Storkey M. *London's Ethnic Minorities: one city, many communities*. London: London Research Centre, 1994; Bardsley M and Morgan D. Deprivation and health in London: an overview of health variations within the capital. *London Journal* 1997; 22:142–59; Anderson H and Flatley J. *Contrasting London incomes: a social and spatial analysis*. London: London Research Centre, 1997.
2. Home Office. *Asylum Statistics 1997*. London: Home Office, 1998.
3. Rounded figures taken as a guide from Storkey M. *London's Ethnic Minorities: one city, many communities*. London: London Research Centre, 1994
4. Home Office. *Asylum Statistics 1997*. London: Home Office, 1998.
5. London Research Centre. *London Housing Statistics 1997*. London: London Research Centre, 1998.
6. Refugee Council. *Factfile Numbers 1–6*, June 1997.
7. Mocroft I, Pharoah C and Romney-Alexander D. *Healthy Relationships: a survey of London health authorities' and trusts' support to the voluntary sector*. Kent: Charities Aid Foundation, 1999.

3. Users' perspectives

This section highlights the key issues from the focus groups with service users. It represents perspectives from 152 service users across London's boroughs. With one exception, all the individuals who participated were contacted through the organisations that responded to the questionnaire. In selecting participants we aimed to get a balance between settled black and minority ethnic communities and more recently arrived refugees and asylum seekers. A profile of the users involved is shown in the second part of Appendix 3. The topic guide for the groups included questions to generate a discussion on why people needed health advocacy support, what they expected to get from advocacy and what standards they expected, whether or not it was important for the advocate or advocacy agency to be independent, and their views on an ideal service.

3.1 Why and how advocacy has been useful

The users who attended the focus groups described their need for advocacy as being associated with:

- gaining basic access to health and social care services
- providing ongoing support to make the best and most effective use of services, particularly in the case of people who used sickle cell and thalassaemia services, mental health services and HIV/AIDS services.

Users across all the care and age groups who participated in the focus groups indicated that they had a need for advocacy support. Users were unanimous in their perceptions that the advocacy support they received helped them to feel more confident about using services and, consequently, to get more out of their service. Many people indicated that as a result of using advocates they no longer felt as timid as they used to, even when they had to attend an appointment without an advocate.

Other studies looking in more detail at users' perspectives of advocacy services have found similar views among users. For example, the MORI[***] study in east London reported that 93 per cent of users surveyed reported feeling more confident when seeing a GP or nurse when they were with an advocate.

The group of users with the most immediate and pressing needs for advocacy support were those who had recently arrived in the UK and whose first language was not English, for example Eastern Europeans and Africans. Many recent arrivals, in particular some Eastern Europeans, did not have the benefit of turning to established communities for the social and moral support that many other groups took for granted. Many indicated that they had experienced hostility and intolerance from individuals within the local communities in which they were placed.

Many people from more established communities, for example Chinese, Vietnamese, Filipino and Latin American communities, identified with that lack of understanding about how services worked, and how this made it necessary to rely on friends, family and local community agencies for advocacy support when using services. This was particularly true for elders from groups such as the Chinese and Vietnamese communities, many of whom had come to the UK late in life and did not speak English.

Receiving advocacy from community organisations was critical for these groups as the community development and infrastructure support advocates offered often played an important role in their lives, as explained by one user:

> *We come to this centre every week because we can see other people from our own community and we can speak our own language and understand each other. Without this centre we would all be very isolated and wouldn't know what to do. We can't rely on our children for everything – we want to be independent as well. The service here is excellent and we are very grateful for it.* (Vietnamese user, Lambeth)

People who were experiencing long-term illnesses such as HIV/AIDS and mental illness underlined how their vulnerability from being ill was compounded by prejudice and discrimination. Many people felt unable to speak up for themselves if they felt uncomfortable

---

[***] MORI. *Evaluation of bi-lingual health advocacy schemes in East London. Evaluation conducted for East London Consortium*. London: MORI, 1994.

with or wanted to disagree with their service provider. In the majority of instances, users highlighted how they relied on the advocacy support provided by a local community organisation or service provider.

Many younger participants (under the age of 20) also identified a need to use advocates. For these young people, who had knowledge of the system and spoke perfect English, their need was less to do with articulating views or access to services than with getting support to deal with the negative impact of racism and discrimination. Their key concern was to have organisations they could trust, as was explained by one participant:

> *Some white girls on my road were throwing stones at my house and when we called the police they said, 'it's not your country, it's their country', so I called the Red Sea Community project for help.* (Service user, Brent)

Users pointed out that black and minority ethnic community organisations offering collective advocacy were often in a unique position to support them in dealing with racism, as was explained by another young person:

> *Racism is more indirect and subtle these days and that's why I think if you have links with a community project, you feel less vulnerable and they can give you the confidence to deal with it as well as to help you out.* (Service user, Harrow)

Language barriers

For newly arrived refugees and asylum seekers, language barriers and a lack of knowledge about how the health and social care system worked were the greatest obstacles. Many felt that if they could speak English properly they would be in a better position to take advantage of any opportunities that existed and to challenge poor practice:

> *Discrimination and prejudice would be easier to deal with if we could at least put our case forward, but we have to rely on someone to speak for us.* (Iranian user, Hammersmith)

More established and settled communities highlighted similar issues, although many people from these groups regularly used the support of friends and families to interpret and translate for them and relied less on individual community agencies and charities. Nevertheless, many users cited examples of when they were simply unable to get basic needs met because of a lack of language support. As one user indicated:

> *I have often been in situations when I haven't been able to find anyone who speaks Farsi and I can't take family members as it's too embarrassing for my son to get involved in explaining what my gynaecological problems are and what I want.* (Iraqi user, Enfield)

Dealing with discrimination and prejudice

A number of users had experiences of service providers who did not want to listen to their needs. Many of the worst experiences users had were of primary care services. For many refugees and asylum seekers who had recently arrived, these experiences compounded the anxieties and stress they experienced from being refugees. Below are some examples given by users:

> *GPs are very unsympathetic towards us. I expect the highest level of support from GPs – I get the opposite.* (Iraqi user, Hammersmith)

> *Sometimes they want to just ignore you and it doesn't matter what you do.* (Somali user, Haringey)

> *My doctor ignored me and I ended up getting pneumonia.* (South American user, Wandsworth)

> *When I go to my GP on my own, he just starts writing the prescription for my tablets, when I take my daughter, he actually listens and that's why I always try and take my daughter, because I know I will get a good service then.* (Greek Cypriot woman, Enfield)

> *I kept going to my doctor because of my pain and he said to me, 'I don't know what your problem is, go home and stay there'. I now have another GP.* (African Caribbean user, Wandsworth)

In a focus group with Kosovan women, the women recounted an experience where some of them had taken their children to register at a GP practice. They went in a group so they would feel safer and more confident. One of the children was found writing on the wall with a crayon and the receptionist asked the whole group to leave, without registering them. The individual recounting the incident said:

> *We felt like we were trash because we were refugees. We don't think they would have thrown us out if we were not refugees.* (Kosovan users, Bromley)

Helping to understand rights and receive entitlements to services

Most people with disabilities or other health needs expressed the need for someone to help them to get their entitlements to services:

> *Sometimes I go to the housing office and they just ignore me – I can speak English, but they don't listen, so many times I go there, I know I have a thick accent, but when I take someone from the project they don't ignore me anymore.* (African user, Lambeth)

> *In July 1997, I found out my daughter was deaf and I needed a lot of help from the project. I felt very lost and bewildered and was trying to come to terms with it as well as trying to get the right services. My daughter is now in school and has started to speak normally. But even now I have contacted social services lots of times to get a hearing loop for her. At first they said yes, then later they said I'm still an asylum seeker and don't know how long I will be here and it's very expensive, I have been many times, but nothing has happened and I know my daughter can't hear even with a hearing aid, and I feel she could pick up much more at home if we had a loop.* (African user, Lambeth)

Providing reassurance and support in an alien environment

Many refugee groups highlighted concerns about being alone and isolated. Many did not have the social support networks that settled and indigenous groups took for granted. The sense of isolation was compounded when people were ill, as was the case within many of the people we spoke with.

Support groups provided a vital link for communities to redevelop relationships and ties within a particular community. Many people offered each other support as 'peer advocates' – especially when there was no other source of support. However, for many people it was equally difficult to seek support from close relatives or friends who were in a similar predicament.

> *It really helped me being with others who had just arrived into the country and were in the same situation – we could get support from each other.* (Chilean user, Wandsworth)

A number of users stated that they felt more comfortable with an advocate who understood and shared their own culture:

> *I still travel from Hammersmith to Alperton and see the GP there because I know that Mrs X is there and she understands my culture and language.* (Somali user, Hammersmith)

Support in learning long-term skills

Many refugees and asylum seekers particularly valued the support organisations provided to meet not only their immediate needs for advocacy but also to enable them to develop long-term skills to help them settle in, find employment and increase their independence. Most people felt that the role that organisations played in helping them move towards greater 'self-advocacy' was critical. One user highlighted her experience of using the Windmill Project in Clapham, which works with refugees and asylum seekers:

I learned skills in computing through the project and they introduced me to English classes so that I could become more independent. (African user living in Lambeth)

3.2 Standards that are important to users

Agreements with advocates

Some users described the process they had gone through with their advocate before meeting service providers as a very important step in building a relationship:

The worker talked to me about what I wanted, how she should represent me, all my housing problems and we agreed what we should say first – it's not lying, but sometimes it matters what you say first. (African user living in Wandsworth)

Advocates who are trained

The majority of users wanted advocates who were trained and had knowledge of relevant legislation, statutory procedures, health, social care and welfare services.

This was particularly important to users working with bi-lingual advocates:

I've had experience of some people who do the job just as soon as they learn a little English and once I got help and my form was filled in incorrectly and now I'm stuck in one place, as I only get a certain level of housing benefit, because of what was written on my form. (Iranian service user living in Barnet)

Confidentiality

There was a consensus that confidentially being upheld by the advocate and the agency was essential. This was linked to the advocate fostering a sense of confidence and demonstrating that he or she was trustworthy and reliable. It was particularly important to users of mental health and HIV services:

We don't want our information being spread around. (African service user living in Haringey)

Advocates who understand users' culture and religion, and who speak the same language

People wanted advocates who understand their situation and problems. For most people their ideal was an advocate from their own community and cultural background who could empathise and represent their interests, and communicate more easily with them.

Advocates who are non-judgemental, assertive and reliable

For a number of users, in particular those of mental health and HIV services, reliability, trustworthiness and being non-judgemental were essential qualities for advocates. All users wanted advocates that were able to empathise with their health concerns and speak up confidently for their needs, especially when they were feeling vulnerable.

3.3 What would users' ideal service provide?

Many users appreciated and were grateful for the services they had received from the organisations we visited. Very often they had not experienced any other models of service provision, which would have allowed them a more objective insight regarding what they might want in an ideal world. Many were unaware of the constraints community organisations worked within.

Most people preferred to describe in a general sense the features of the service that they used or wanted most, rather than isolating specific aspects. However, there were a number of practical ideas mentioned – many of which reiterated the standards described below.

Service availability

Most people wanted a service that would be available when they needed it and not when it suited the service provider. Many people who used sickle cell and HIV services felt strongly about this. People said they were at their most vulnerable during periods when the services were closed, at night and during weekends. Many people felt that access during out-of-hours periods should be made easier, for example by providing a telephone link that was available for 24 hours each day, particularly at weekends.

A service that works across statutory and voluntary sector boundaries

There was consensus among users across all groups that an advocate should be able to work with them in any situation or with any of the services that they used. The advocate should offer a 'one-stop' service and help guide them through the system, as for many health, housing and social care needs were inextricably linked.

Service location

Most people wanted a service that was easy to get to, but they did not place too great an importance on this. In general, people visited a local service where they received support from the staff in that agency. For individual cases, advocates would often travel to where the client needed to meet a service provider or where they lived.

Continuity of service provision

Continuity of contact with service provider organisations and an advocate was very important for most service users. Many favoured a community development approach to not only meeting immediate support needs (as they were isolated, and felt vulnerable) but also because they had experienced the advocacy service as positive and empowering and wanted to build on it to help themselves more, as well as to help others:

> *I prefer one person to deal with, then you don't have to start from scratch each time and sometimes it can be painful to explain.* (Iranian service user living in Barnet)

> *It would be great if we could have a drop-in here and after-schools places.* (Somali user living in Harrow)

> *We would like to meet here everyday and not just a Thursday as we are on our own at home.* (Greek Cypriot user living in Enfield)

Independent service or not?

Service users expressed both indifference and concern about whether the advocate was independent or not. In general, users who were less familiar with the system and relied very heavily on the support of advocates expressed very few opinions on this issue and generally did not seem to care.

> *To me it doesn't matter really – it's just because we know this service.* (Kosovan user living in Bromley)

Others users, especially young people, from communities that were well-established in the UK and who were long-term service users, had particular views that, to a large extent, correlated with the type of advocacy support they had positive experiences of. For example, people who used a hospital linkworker scheme felt it was very important for advocates to be based as part of the service because then they felt they were better able to help; they saw the linkworkers as part of the larger organisation and felt they were accepted and respected by the staff. Others, particularly people who used mental health, HIV/AIDS and sickle cell services, were suspicious of advocates provided by service providers and felt that such a service should be independent so that the advocate did not collude with staff:

> *Sometimes, especially in hospitals, they can all stick together or cover things up and close ranks.* (Greek Cypriot user living in Enfield)

4. Themes for developing advocacy services in London

This section identifies the key themes emerging from the study on which future actions can be developed. It draws together the key issues arising from the questionnaires, in-depth interviews, focus group discussions with service providers, funders and trainers and the reference group,[†††] to provide a fuller understanding of the findings of this study.

While a number of important themes have emerged from the study, we have been cautious about interpreting some results where we had a low response and which were solely reliant on quantitative data. When we felt there was an important issue and the data was limited or was not collected by the survey we have cross-referred to other related research in this area to support any conclusions drawn.

Throughout this section we use illustrative quotes taken from focus group discussions and interviews to add richness and reality to the issues highlighted. Practical, real life examples are used to showcase good practice and provide examples of what can be achieved.

4.1 Mainstreaming advocacy

Many providers felt that advocacy should be a 'core' element of delivering services in London, where there is such wide diversity and disadvantage. One provider commented:

> *Advocacy is a service that should be provided strategically ... to remedy inequality and discrimination, and to develop more user-focused care and greater community and user involvement.*

There was a strong perception that advocacy services lacked investment and were not recognised or valued sufficiently within health and social care settings. This was attributed to low value associated with *user empowerment* and *choice*, a lack of awareness among many

[†††] Appendix 3 provides a summary of all the sources from which these issues have been collated. All focus group meetings were recorded and transcribed for accuracy and consistency. The contents of all reference group meetings and interviews were based on flipchart and hand-written notes. The issues that emerged from questionnaire responses were recorded 'verbatim' on the database.

managers and professionals about advocacy roles, and a lack of empirical evidence on the added value and cost benefits that advocacy may offer to service users.

Most agencies identified the negative perceptions of many managers and professionals within statutory agencies as a significant barrier to the development and acceptance of advocacy within mainstream health and social care services. The fact that people who tend to use advocacy services are among the most vulnerable and discriminated-against groups in society placed 'advocacy development' within statutory agencies as a low priority, which offered little attraction for career development for managers and professionals alike:

> *The nature of advocacy is that we deal with people who are very much on the margins ... who are discriminated against. They're a group of clients that don't have a high profile, that are not able to look out for themselves. There are real issues around advocates wanting to raise and highlight the needs of this client (BME) base. I think there are real issues around institutional racism.*

> *Our project works a lot with asylum seekers. The general climate for asylum seekers has really deteriorated ... so it's an uphill struggle. We are working in a climate where the needs of our clients are not generally recognised. There is a tension between what we are trying to do and what is going on in the wider field.*

More than half the agencies in the study identified poor receptiveness of statutory agencies as a fundamental issue. Tension between advocacy providers and statutory agencies was described as common, which most agencies related to a limited understanding and acceptance of advocacy by statutory agencies.

> *It's a point of friction sometimes, because the advocates try to get better services from the provider, so the provider can get a little bit touchy about the advocate.*

There was an equally strong perception among agencies that statutory professionals often resented the role of advocates, which was seen as interfering, threatening or unnecessary. While professionals' perceptions of advocacy were beyond the scope of the study, there is useful research[1] showing that certain professionals regard third party involvement in client–professional relationships as undermining, as it changes the power dynamic between the professional and client. For some, the acknowledgement that a client may need an advocate implied criticism of their ability to meet the clients' needs and was seen as an admission of failure. This perspective contrasts with other studies, which show hospital doctors positively welcoming the intervention of bi-lingual advocates.[2]

There is clearly a need for greater clarity and understanding about the role of advocates vis-à-vis encouraging empowerment, and choice and about the advocacy role that many professionals in the NHS and social services will undertake in the course of their work with clients. These roles, though different, are not in conflict but, rather, are complementary, and it is important to realise that the advocacy role of a clinician or social worker can often conflict with the interests of the service user.

The Government's modernisation agenda places fast, fair and convenient services at the heart of its national strategy to improve health and social services. Empowerment and choice for service users are highlighted as being key to the delivery of user-centred services. There are a range of initiatives and directives that provide significant opportunities to develop services that begin to place what the user wants and needs as priorities. These strategic shifts in national policy now provide a more favourable environment to promote and develop advocacy services.

4.2 Strategic co-ordination and improved networking

The need for a co-ordinating agency or forum for advocacy workers was identified by two-thirds of agencies as a strategic priority for developing services. Many wanted to see a dedicated network that would encourage the strategic development of health advocacy services for black and minority ethnic communities, promote the sharing of good practice and learning, and raise awareness and promote a more acceptable image of advocacy across health and social care sectors.

The process of developing a network would need to ensure that small organisations were actively encouraged to participate and not just dominated by larger, better resourced and experienced agencies.

While most agencies agreed that an agency or network should be established to assist in the promotion, co-ordination and development of advocacy, views about its organisation and structure were less well defined. General caution was also expressed with regard to resourcing such a venture on a short-term basis, which could easily raise expectations that would be difficult to fulfil without sustainable funding.

A number of important benefits of developing a network were described:

- **It would help strategic development.** For many agencies, the strategic development of advocacy was critical to break cycles of reinventing 'the issues' or being 'in vogue'. For example, many felt that advocacy was now 'flavour of the month' as a result of national initiatives to promote involvement and participation and increase choice for users, and development was seen as an opportunity that should be taken now.

- **A forum could play a strategic role** in campaigning for better policies, resources and development of advocacy services on a pan-London and national level. This would help to keep the issue of advocacy alive and on Government agendas:

  Advocacy has got to assert itself in the extent to how well established it is. I think one of the problems that we've got is that advocacy providers are so small and we have to be like small little spiders all doing their own thing, all duplicating each other's work, all remaining, you know, in terms of organisational structure, very simple structures. We have to move on from there ... I'd like to see more organisational managers, more structure created, better established organisations so we don't have to continually justify ourselves, and perhaps do loads of research to justify our existence. We can just be and develop. (Focus group participant)

- **It would create a structure to share ideas, good practice and learning.** Many saw the main value of a forum as providing a structure where workers could meet to develop and refine their ideas and methods of working. Most agencies highlighted the fact that there are very few opportunities for practitioners to discuss and debate issues in a constructive and positive environment.

- **It would provide opportunities, directly and indirectly, for better networking among health advocates.** Many providers felt that advocates themselves often had little opportunity for development, sharing experiences and ideas relating to their work:

Advocacy would really benefit from having a strong voice in an organised way, if there was a way of bringing together people ... I was really excited by being invited and wanted to find out who the other people in the other focus groups were, I wanted to talk to them. (Focus group participant)

- **It would enhance the status of advocacy.** Many providers felt that advocacy suffered from low status and credibility among many managers and professionals. A forum could help co-ordinate and maximise efforts to educate and raise awareness.

- **It could co-ordinate and broker services.** Many providers are restricted in their capacity due to economies of scale and many find it difficult to respond to the increasingly diverse demands of service users in London. A co-ordinating agency could develop and maintain an active database of providers, particularly of those who could provide some of the less common languages at short notice and could manage and broker services and skills – services that are in high demand but short supply:

  We have found ... being a small organisation, that networking with other small organisations is similar to the blind leading the blind – none of us know anything!

- **It should be led by black and minority ethnic communities.** A common theme raised by many providers was that a network in this field working for black and minority ethnic communities needed to be led by black and minority ethnic communities:

  We need to a provide a forum for minority ethnic communities to set their own agenda.

  There should be a black and ethnic minority consortium run by black groups, not a white institution.

- **It should build on existing networks rather than create new ones.** There were also views that the emphasis needed to be on building the strengths and efforts of existing advocacy networks in London rather than creating new ones. Our review of current networks in Appendix 11 shows that these networks tend to be client- and care group-focused and do not specifically address issues for black and minority ethnic communities and workers within their work programmes.

4.3 Assessing impact and standards

The analysis in Section 2 indicated that very few outcome-focused measures were used. Many providers indicated that the key to successfully mainstreaming and developing advocacy was for advocacy agencies to collectively adopt a more assertive stance and move from a position of constantly justifying the need for advocacy. Some agencies felt that 'core standards' would clearly help them to become more accepted and to legitimise their role, which in turn would benefit their clients. Others highlighted the dangers of professionalising advocacy, which they felt would work against small black organisations:

> *Once you professionalise it, it becomes elitist and exclusive rather than inclusive.*

Another focus for standards came from the perspectives of users. The areas identified are covered in greater detail in Section 3. They are summarised in the table below:

Table 4.1: Standards for advocacy providers

Standards relating to the advocate
1. Advocates should establish an agreement with the client before meeting the service providers to explain the advocate's role and build a relationship
2. Advocates should be trained and have knowledge of relevant legislation, statutory procedures, health, social care and welfare services
3. The relationship between the advocate and client should be strictly confidential. This was a particular concern to users of mental health and HIV services and for many refugee groups. A study in 1995 in south London found that a number of refugees believed that their GP worked for the Home Office![3]
4. Advocates should understand the culture and religion of, and speak the same language as, the client
5. Advocates should be non-judgemental, assertive and reliable
Standards relating to the service provided
1. Services should be available beyond normal office hours and at weekends
2. A telephone link that should be available 24 hours a day and particularly at weekends
3. The service should provide support across statutory and voluntary sector boundaries
4. Services should be easy to get to
5. Services should provide continuity of contact with the client as far as possible
6. The relationship between the agency and client should be strictly confidential

Funders agreed that small and low funded advocacy services could not have the same impact as larger organisations. Thus, in terms of developing standards of effectiveness, for example, there was consensus that funders needed to adjust their criteria accordingly. There were a number of funders and providers who agreed that advocacy agencies needed to develop more objective ways to monitor and assess the needs of their clients in order to demonstrate their effectiveness and develop stronger business cases.

The model shown in Appendix 12 was developed with the Project Reference Group in an attempt to define the features of basic monitoring which *all* providers could reasonably be expected to adopt, progressing to areas that would add value in assessing the effectiveness and impact of the service provided.

The focus group and reference group discussions on the 'effectiveness' of advocacy services and how it could be measured provided further insights to complement questionnaire responses on the practices and experiences of providers and funders.

There was consensus from all groups that effectiveness should be addressed at a strategic planning level as well as at the point of service delivery if it was to be demonstrated in any evaluation of the service. A balance between objective and subjective methods was seen as necessary, not only to assess outputs and outcomes but also to capture the experiences of clients to get a 'real' insight into the impact and added value of the service. User feedback was seen as providing a valuable insight into the way services were provided and what changes were needed.

Key elements of the criteria to measure effectiveness that emerged from the cross-section of respondents are combined within the table overleaf.

Table 4.2: Framework for assessing effectiveness

Area for assessment	*Assessment criteria/measures*
1. Evidence of appropriate systems for monitoring and evaluation of the service	Systems of basic data collection and monitoring of the service provided in terms of numbers of clients seen, client feedback, financial accountability and control; basic services delivery standards, e.g. waiting and response times
2. How the provider empowers service users	Information provided as part of the process; identifying the type of support given; providing publicity and information; making appropriate referrals
3. Evidence of minimising the negative impact of cultural barriers	Awareness of clients about services, care and treatment; awareness of professionals about clients cultural and religious needs; effective communication between clients and service providers
4. How the provider achieves a user-led service	Involvement of users in planning, management and decision-making
5. How the provider promotes access to relevant procedures and mechanisms for communication and feedback	Complaints procedures and feedback systems of external organisations
6. Evidence of user accountability and confidentiality	Evidence of relevant procedures and reporting such as annual reports and AGMs
7. User feedback of experience of the advocacy service	Complaints, anecdotal feedback and user surveys
8. Evidence of change in the organisation and at the point of service delivery	Evidence that care plans are influenced/supported; appropriate use of A&E; uptake rates; demand on GP consultations; patients' health and quality of life; other positive impact measures, such as greater involvement of users in consultations
9. Evidence of growth and development within the service	Staff training and development programmes
10. How the service reduces inequalities	Measures of long-term impact on, e.g. clients' ability to make better and informed choices, to access and use services to achieve personal goals

4.4 Cross-sector working

The realities of people's lives mean that agencies often handle situations that straddle health, social care, welfare and housing issues. This was evident from the experiences of the majority of agencies and from the expectations of service users. While there are a small number of dedicated advocacy providers that only work with NHS clients, the large majority of agencies located in the voluntary sector work across all care sectors, mirroring the needs and demands of their clients.

The way in which many agencies operate reflects how their links and relationships with the statutory agencies that they were assisting clients to use, were less that ideal and in some cases quite poor. Those advocacy providers that were based within NHS organisations had, as expected, good local links within the organisation as they were regarded as part of the services provided by the trust. However, few others reported good all round links. In fact, a common theme emerging for independent advocacy providers, that is those not based in the statutory sector, was the difficulty in establishing the necessary links and relationships to maintain the provision of effective services. While it was not measured, many agencies indicated that enormous time and energy went into managing relationships when they felt that this time could otherwise have been spent on developing and providing services.

Generic providers tended to have links with a wider range of agencies and most appeared to be linked into some local network of voluntary groups or advocacy agencies, although advocacy networks were identified far less frequently. The exception was for the smaller agencies that had three or less paid members of staff, which identified that they generally had poor or no links with any local networks.

Overall, agencies felt they had the poorest links with Community Health Councils and Racial Equality Councils. This may be an area that should be examined further, given the 'health' and 'black and minority ethnic' focus of the study and the important local role that both these types of agencies play as 'formal' advocates for users. Poor links were also highlighted with the primary care sector generally. However, we have to take into account the fact that the research took place when primary care groups were still developing and would not have had the infrastructure in place to reflect the types of links anticipated. The importance of primary care providers has, however, been highlighted previously with regard to the gate-keeping role of GPs (see Section 1.7).

Users expressed very clearly that they preferred to use services that could assist them in dealing with all care agencies they had contact with, as their basic need for using any service was similar. Many health advocacy agencies acknowledged this. As one provider pointed out:

You can't tell people to go away if they come with a domestic violence case or housing issues.

4.5 Independent advocacy or not?

One of the philosophical dilemmas to emerge was the issue of whether advocacy services should be completely independent of mainstream service providers or whether they could operate just as effectively as a part of larger organisations, as some of the advocacy providers in the study actually do. Different organisations were clearly practising in a similar fashion but with different philosophical and political understandings of 'the nature of advocacy'.

A number of agencies felt it was appropriate to provide advocacy support as part of a wider range of services offered, to complement and enhance access to the services they provided (for example linking it directly to health promotion and outreach work or to interpreting services). Many of these agencies did not have fixed or dogmatic views about the nature of advocacy, beyond that it was 'a good thing' and that it 'benefited' service users. This position accounted for the majority of agencies who responded to the questionnaire. Others felt that an advocacy service could only be truly effective if the community that it served managed it. This understanding is much more closely aligned to fundamental principles of user-led services, which guide the work of many organisations:

My group has been set up to provide an independent advocacy service, for the simple reason that the main provision of advocacy services in Camden and Islington are provided by the bodies which we are advocating for or against. Obviously there are agendas in providing these services by the statutory bodies anyway. There are some difficulties which we've encountered in practice, with some people coming along and saying, 'I am employed by this health authority as an advocate and I will advocate for you' and some job descriptions actually say that the advocate cannot get involved in a case against the employing authority.

A number of providers in the focus groups felt it was important that advocacy providers did not take up polarised positions in this debate. While some agencies felt a clear philosophical position was important, as a principle and for the integrity of the service, others did not feel as strongly. There are nevertheless merits to both sides of the argument.

NHS trust-based health advocacy providers highlighted some of the benefits of being a part of an NHS trust. These were the ease with which they developed relationships with trust staff and departments, being regarded as colleagues and part of trust services, a clear rationale for raising awareness about the services provided, and automatic links to internal mechanisms and structures for channelling feedback obtained from patients.

A drawback identified by a number of NHS trust advocates was managing situations where the interests of the client placed them in conflict with the trust or a clinician. A number of advocates indicated that many clinicians expected advocates to support them, as they were both trust employees and, more often than not, the clinician was in the senior position.

Independent, voluntary sector-based health advocacy providers felt very strongly about the principle of not compromising their independent status and highlighted the fact that their loyalties were clearly with the patient. The majority had high levels of user participation within the service or were user-led.

Drawbacks highlighted were difficulties in developing links and relationships with statutory providers, not being taken seriously as a 'proper' service and poor referrals to their service. These drawbacks, while inconvenient and time consuming, were generally accepted as 'par for the course' and tackled within the work programme to raise awareness and build links.

Merits of other models

All the statutory sector-based advocacy providers explained how their location and status as part of an NHS trust had enabled them to nurture relationships within the trust and gain acceptance of their service:

> *To make any change you need to have advocacy but you also need other systems to tap into. It's not one or the other but complementing and working with them. In our case we are completely independent, we have very clear service protocols, but at the same time we know that we are actually speaking for clients and even if the consultants say, 'I don't need you', we don't actually agree to that. We will go if the client needs us. We insist on being there if the client wants us.*

Another perspective on the value of statutory sector advocacy was that there is easier access to resources to develop the service:

> *In the voluntary sector there aren't supportive management and training structures at the moment for advocacy to survive there.*

Some anxiety was expressed about applying a rigid compact to streamline and develop advocacy in one way. The needs of the black and minority ethnic communities in question should always be paramount:

> *We shouldn't say there's one model or another because we feel very strongly that there were benefits from being part of the system. What makes our service effective is that we've been incorporated into a multidisciplinary team and accepted to such an extent that we are equal partners in the process and not being excluded. That might not be appropriate, I think in mental health it probably isn't appropriate, it's a different kind of service. It might be idealistic, so you've got to build in safeguards and protocols.*

This debate will develop as work continues. Our guidance at this stage is for the agencies that lead the development of this work to facilitate unbiased and open discussion. The litmus test for services contemplating the issue of 'independence' should be the question 'are we user-led or not?' There appears to be scope and need for a range of approaches that can appropriately serve the needs of the many different communities in London:

> *In Hackney there is a very large Turkish community. A community organisation providing advocacy would be very well used. In Newham, we have a lot of very small communities who haven't actually got community organisations, who benefit from the Trust actually taking on the responsibility to provide an advocate. I think we mustn't lose sight of that, because the onus of providing advocacy needs to be on the provider rather than the health service user. I think people can only benefit from that.*

4.6 Developing small providers

A number of advocacy providers, large and small, recognised the need for and the value of the work that small black and minority ethnic organisations were doing:

My own experience is, any project that has been successful with black people is a small one where black people can work with black people.

Many minority ethnic groups/organisations are usually made of committed individuals who through life experiences decided to help others. Lack of appropriate funding for these groups usually affects their development and performance. Attention is always focused on mainstream providers or bigger organisations. However these smaller organisations are full of dedicated individuals that can make a difference to peoples' lives.

However, the ability of many of these organisations to grow and develop or even provide a quality service is questionable when a large number of them have no or very few funded staff. These organisations can never compete with larger agencies for limited resources, yet many of them are lifelines for vulnerable people within their own communities, especially newly arrived refugees and asylum seekers. These groups need to be targeted for support and development to raise them to a level where they can begin to participate and compete.

Developing capacity

Many small organisations recognised that funders should take account of their infrastructure and development needs. This sentiment was also echoed by many of the funding agencies that responded. Some funders identified a range of support and development options, which were offered to organisations that need this type of assistance.

The nature of the work undertaken by small agencies often leads to demands that exceed their capacity. This was described in terms of their management capability, responding to the demands of different communities and the continuous job of fund-raising:

Even if you're working within specific ethnic groups, it's quite often made out that their needs are homogenous, and they're not.

Many agencies indicated that a consequence of balancing excess demand against capability was to provide a basic level of advocacy that just offered clients enough to get by rather than being able to fully represent them all the way through:

> *Our clients are mainly refugees and asylum seekers. They are in great need of advocates. The form of advocacy we are providing, I would say, is really primitive. If we're honest, we are just providing interpreters rather than professional advocates.*

Many black and minority ethnic organisations felt that they lacked credibility with large providers because of their size. This highlights the need for raising awareness and training for statutory agencies to better understand and appreciate the roles and contributions that small organisations make, and to make efforts to improve working relationships:

> *One of the problems we have is that if you come from a big organisation and you come to a hospital, people give you a lot of co-operation. If you are a volunteer from a small community organisation probably you don't get their respect. So this has a lot of effect on our volunteers.*

Invisibility was an area that concerned a number of newer communities, such as Armenians and even some more settled communities like the Vietnamese. While groups such as the Vietnamese have coped with being dispersed and isolated, they still feel that they do not have strong representation for issues that are specific to their communities. Newer groups like Armenians suffer from a type of 'cultural sterilisation'. There is no ethnic category within the current ONS classifications for Armenians, a problem compounded by the fact that many Armenians arrive in the UK from different countries. In the absence of any useful classification they are incorrectly recorded as 'white British':

> *One of the specific problems that Armenians face in comparison with other minority and refugee communities is that they are 'invisible'. This is why advocacy is so important to Armenians. Armenian as an ethnic group is not defined in the ONS Census classifications. Many arrive from different countries, therefore local authorities, hospitals and GPs often record their nationalities as 'British' or only their country of birth. Consequently, their specific social, health and cultural needs are not generally recognised or addressed by the statutory or voluntary sector agencies. This lack of awareness about who Armenians are and where they are from reinforces the alienation felt by the 20,000 Armenians living in London.*

Retaining volunteers was also a key theme to emerge, particularly in the focus groups with small organisations that did not provide advocacy as a main part of their service. The majority of these indicated that they were dependent on unpaid staff to provide the advocacy support they offered to clients.

One organisation related their experience of the barriers they encountered in trying to retain volunteers:

> *We had 15 volunteers in the middle of last year. From those 15 persons, we have now only five. It is very difficult to keep them. For example, when they come from central London to Earl's Court, they need transport, and they need £5.00 for lunch. So if you don't have that amount of money, it's difficult. We do have people who clearly want to help the community and if they know they will get some training, and in the future some employment, that would help.*

4.7 Issues for bi-lingual advocacy

A current issue of confusion and debate, which often results in a poorer service for the client, is the accepted need to distinguish interpreting and advocacy as separate functions. Many agencies that provide interpreting services also see themselves as advocacy providers, while others do not. Often it is simply inconsistency with the use of the descriptive terms used, for example, as we described in Section 1, many terms such as 'linkworker', 'advocate' and 'interpreter' are used interchangeably to describe roles with different fundamental functions. Most agencies accept the simplistic distinction discussed in Section 1 to highlight the essential difference between advocacy and interpreting:

An interpreter finds out from the client the answers to the staff's questions and relays to the client the staff's wishes or directives.

An advocate finds out from the staff the answers to the patient's questions and communicates the client's wishes.

Further elaboration on these roles show that the key role of an interpreter is to provide impartial communication or negotiation, not to represent the interests of either party in the process. His or her role is to 'encode' messages and information from the service provider to the service user and vice-versa. The interpreter often provides a specific service that is confined to communicating with a service provider and user at a specific point in time. The advocate, on the other hand, is solely concerned with the needs and wishes of the client, working in a proactive manner to defined outcomes that help the service user to achieve their rights and obtain the very best from services. The model shown in Appendix 13 was developed by a service provider in London to illustrate the different roles of advocates, linkworkers and interpreters.

While these definitions are helpful, there is not yet an overarching academic framework in which to ground these definitions or sufficient practitioners adhering to a common code of practice to establish them as everyday practices. Other studies carried out reveal that advocacy practices vary considerably, as do the levels of skill and competence of advocates. Equally, the training opportunities available to advocates are often inadequate.[4]

This lack of clarity has created difficulties for bi-lingual service providers seeking contracts, for example where commissioners have stipulated the purchase of interpreting and not advocacy services. A number of bi-lingual advocacy providers with substantial expertise in this field start with assessing the need of the clients as their first priority. If advocacy support is required while carrying out interpreting (which it often is) then that is also provided – with very clear explanations offered to the professional about the role of the interpreter/advocate.

Some white organisations acknowledged difficulties in trying to access bi-lingual advocates. Many black organisations felt that some white organisations were not handling properly the recruitment of advocates to work with bi-lingual communities:

> *The problem that we face in Newham is we've got mental health advocacy projects but their advocates do not cover diverse languages. So we have a mental health advocate, and a bi-lingual advocate ... so for one group you end up having four people doing an assessment – you have a psychologist, a doctor, a mental health advocate and a bi-lingual advocate!*

4.8 Primary care issues

Many providers highlighted huge areas of unmet need in primary care, particularly within GP practices. Common experiences were of GPs refusing to use advocacy and interpreting services and the lack of understanding of the needs of refugees and new arrivals by primary care workers:

> *The problem for refugees and asylum seekers is that GPs can refuse to register them – that's what's happening. They don't register these patients.*

> *Of 120 GP practices in Camden and Islington there's probably ten that use us and of those about seven use us consistently. It's not because minority ethnic communities are concentrated in those areas, it's because those are the enlightened practices. The big challenge is to get them on board. I've trained receptionists, sent out endless mail, put posters up and still it's the same handful that uses us. I don't know how you overcome that problem.*

> *I've got a number of cases now, from different parts of London. West London ... where GPs are refusing to contact interpreting and advocacy services.*

Some providers indicated that the barriers they faced with GPs were not only confined to the use of advocacy services, but reflected wider inequalities in service delivery at a primary care level:

> *This is actually racism, institutional racism, that needs to be addressed, because GPs are serving a community in a very non-appropriate manner.*

Some organisations, particularly those serving refugee communities, relayed experiences of failed attempts of trying to work proactively with GPs:

> *Many of our clients feel dissatisfied when they go to their GPs. Often they have gone for a second opinion which has turned out to be different. We tried to work with many of these GP practices to provide cultural awareness training. When we contacted them the GPs didn't want it, yet we know there is a problem. We feel they are denying that they have a need to understand more about these refugee groups.*

There were a number of positive examples in primary care where practitioners were working with local groups to develop more responsive services. An evaluation of health access for black and minority ethnic communities undertaken in 1999[5] indicated that a number of primary care groups had identified issues relating to access, equality and diversity within local priorities. However, as highlighted in Section 2, primary care management is undergoing radical structural changes and, while this presents some upheaval, there are likely to be positive benefits relating to how primary care groups work with GP practices and local community groups to develop more sensitive local services and improve access.

4.9 Funding issues

Provider perspectives

Investing in advocacy. The sourcing and availability of funding for advocacy services is an area that concerns the majority of agencies that responded. However, it is difficult to draw conclusions here regarding how appropriate the current level of investment indicated is and also what it should be, as that data is not available through this survey or elsewhere. Wider comparisons would also have to be made against the overall level of investment in such work within the voluntary sector as a whole (which is where the vast majority of these agencies are located), which was beyond the scope of this survey.

Recent research into the level of spending across London in the voluntary sector by major funders points to lower than average levels of spending within black and minority ethnic communities compared to their representation within the population. The research pointed to about 2.9 per cent of health spending in the voluntary sector going to black and minority ethnic agencies.[‡‡‡]

What is clear is that the majority of black and minority ethnic projects are funded on a short-term basis, which severely restricts their ability to make any significant impact or to achieve real growth and development.

Fund-raising expertise. Many small agencies felt disadvantaged as they had no dedicated staff with specific fund-raising skills to negotiate and re-negotiate contracts and complete funding proposals. Often they felt that funding applications did not match the expectations or

---

‡‡‡ Mocroft I, Pharoah C and Romney-Alexander D. *Healthy Relationships: a Survey of London health authorities' and trusts' support to the voluntary sector*. Kent: Charities Aid Foundation, 1999.

criteria that funders expected. For example, many refugee organisations stated that they often had to respond to crisis situations and needed to find extra resources to meet such demands. This dimension of how they work is often not accommodated within existing contracts.

Many small organisations that were not funded to provide advocacy highlighted a need to improve their knowledge and general skills in fund-raising. Many were starting at a very basic level:

> *I find it very difficult to find sources of statutory funding. I've got to grips with trusts and charities, even the National Lottery, but I don't understand where government funding comes from. I find it very complicated. For instance I really do not know how to access PCGs. Unless I personally go to all the meetings, it's quite hard to know how to use them. Certain names come up in your local borough and you think they are the powerful people – but how do I access these people? You hear the names over and over again and you think, well I don't know them, so it's quite difficult to get at them. It doesn't always feel terribly democratic.*

Fitting in with funding agencies' priorities. Many agencies indicated that they found it burdensome to develop their services in the way they wished to because of short-term funding constraints. Changing funding priorities and requests for 'new' and 'innovative' schemes were seen as another impediment, which forced many agencies to re-shape their proposals in order to re-submit them to match new funding criteria:

> *Every year there are projects that they give £30,000 and every year it's a small organisation you never heard of before. They come up when the grants are there, and then they disappear. They have no effect on the community. What I'd like to see is core funding for some organisations, to build them. Some organisations that are there for a long time might get £2000, compared to £100,000 for a new organisation. It's not fair.*

> *Advocacy is flavour of the month, it is the buzzword at the moment, it's something new, something exciting, and for me the big challenge is how to make it into an accepted part of mainstream health services. I have this great fear that something else will come up and advocacy will slip down to the bottom of the agenda again.*

Accountability of funding agencies. Most agencies felt that funders should also be monitored and their programmes evaluated with feedback provided to communities about what improvements had resulted from their funding strategies and priorities.

Funder perspectives

Capacity building. The majority of funding agencies who responded to the questionnaire highlighted the need for infrastructure development in the black voluntary sector. Particular views were expressed about smaller organisations developing links with and receiving support from larger umbrella organisations, for example through shadowing and mentoring.

Advocacy is a generic activity. Some funders felt that for many of the organisations they funded, health advocacy was often included as part of the larger agenda and workloads, without necessarily being defined as such. This posed a difficulty for them in isolating or quantifying how much of their funding went to support this area of work:

> *Health advocacy is often 'hidden' in generic work.*

Need for clearer definitions. There were a number of suggestions for clearer definitions and outcome criteria to be developed in this area. Some funders also felt that the agencies who applied to them did not fully understand advocacy themselves and often confused it with interpreting.

Measuring the impact of advocacy. The measurement of the long-term impact of health advocacy work was an area where a number of funders wished to see more development. Funders felt that by developing and using more objective and outcome focused criteria for monitoring and evaluation, it would be easier for advocacy service providers to demonstrate the value and benefits of their work to mainstream statutory agencies. This is important when considering that a significant number of funding agencies themselves are mainstream statutory bodies. For example, some funders perceived advocacy as an expensive service to fund and develop, but admitted that they had no evidence or analysis of 'perceived' versus 'real' costs. Many funders had no understanding of the types of services they would need to provide for individuals who did not receive formal advocacy support.

Collaboration among funding agencies. Some funders expressed a need for funders to collaborate. Those who had tried had experienced difficulties working with partner agencies to develop common standards and sustainable funding.

Funders themselves highlighted the issue of developing longer-term funding to voluntary sector organisations. Some funders admitted that without any safeguards it was much easier for them to cut the funding of voluntary sector organisations:

> *The reality is that statutory services are more secure than voluntary sector services and when you have to make cuts and savings, it is much easier to cut voluntary sector rather than carve out something out of statutory services. For example it's virtually impossible to make cuts in London hospitals – easy as pie to make them in the voluntary sector.*

Developing ethnicity monitoring. Some statutory funders in localities with regular arrivals of refugees and asylum seekers indicated that poor ethnic monitoring made it virtually impossible to estimate the volume of services they needed to secure. This was also compounded by the fact that many refugees, asylum seekers and homeless people were more reluctant to provide monitoring information in Census and other local monitoring mechanisms:

> *Accurate knowledge of population size is completely impossible and when the health authority was doing an estimate there was a 10 per cent margin, but when you are already walking on the edge of a cliff as far as funding is concerned 10 per cent quite obviously pushes you over the edge, and because you just cannot manage and we have such a high percentage of immigrants, refugees, asylum seekers and homeless people, they are the ones who are reluctant to report to the Census. Ethnic monitoring is inaccurately carried out so we have a hard time.*

4.10 Training issues

Advocacy provider perspectives

Link training programmes to career development. A number of advocacy providers and agencies providing training wanted to develop training that was part of a *career structure* for advocates:

> *What I'm training is bi-lingual advocates, but basically it's advocacy and there are not too many opportunities for career development. You can always find money for training and endlessly train people. What do they get at the end of it?*

> *One of my concerns for a number of years has been progression, because it is not an organised field of work yet.*

One provider described a method that was based on 'community development' principles to recruit individuals in the area of bereavement services:

> *I think foundation training has to go on to bring skills up in certain communities. Every year we try and recruit people, but some areas, like befriending, require slightly less developed skills, so my idea is that you define the skills in levels and develop people to progress through those levels. For example, when you start with an 18-year-old young woman who can manage befriending in her own community, by the time she's 21 ... she might be ready to do counselling, and from there she might get a psychology degree or a nursing qualification. You can link with local colleges, as many people need experience to get into caring courses ... that's quite important because volunteers can get training in return, and that's how we keep the good volunteers, we train them up.*

A number of organisations identified the importance of setting up training that establishes links with prospective employers to provide an additional incentive and potential opportunity for employment. One organisation described their experience of this:

> *There is a programme in our area; it's called Refugees into Jobs. The main problem is, these people say OK, I'll go on this course for six months – and they don't get*

employed. Most of them are mothers, they have small children. They say, 'I want to better myself. I'm ready to go into that course'. But after six months the refugees aren't better off. And then they question it.

Experiences of training agencies

Designing and developing appropriate courses. Many training agencies underlined how the content, focus, availability and methods of accreditation for their courses were often determined by the priorities of their funding agency. One agency gave an example that affected how they were able to describe their courses:

We get European funding and advocacy as a word is not recognised in Europe, so we have to use the word 'mediation' to be in line with Europe – tends to be called cultural mediation or cross-cultural mediation.

Collaboration with employers. One agency stressed the need for employers and commissioning agencies to be more directly involved in the design and delivery of training. Training agencies often experienced little collaboration from employers over their requirements for job specifications. For example, some agencies described how statutory sector agencies often nominated guest speakers for courses that failed to provide any context about the job requirements of the advocate in their presentations.

Practical work placements to complement training were highlighted as an essential preparation for advocates.

Training for bi-lingual advocates. Training providers had different views about the availability of training for bi-lingual advocates. Where providers felt a gap did not exist they emphasised a need to provide flexible training programmes that identified and developed a learner's skills, as both effective health advocate and effective interpreter within a health advocacy context.

One agency offered community interpreting and advocacy courses as separate modules and highlighted how employers, because of the resource implications, often choose a single module when both are required.

Accreditation and standards. Training agencies recognised the need to achieve standardisation of advocacy training across London and possibly to work towards a national standard. One training provider said:

> *In my experience people come to you from different courses and their knowledge is very different, some of them are not suitable and I usually need to train them again.*

Agencies felt that development of standards needed to be supported by parallel developments to raise awareness about the role of advocacy and advocates with statutory agencies and advocacy providers:

> *[Advocacy] needs at least putting onto the map before you start designing occupational and training structure, otherwise you overload them. It will be down to the person who is being trained at pre-higher education level to manage the communication with a person who has three degrees and does not intend to be managed.*

Agencies felt there was no single route that was best suited to develop accreditation or indeed clarity on what the accreditation standards should be. Three options were highlighted:

- *the Open College system.* The ethos of the Open College system was described by one training body as 'a compromise between being responsive to local situations and to changing situations'. The advantage of this accreditation system identified by many providers was that the accreditation units could be used in other areas, thereby offering a 'currency' for people to progress their education and careers
- *national professional qualification body.* The view on this was that, as a London-wide organisation has not been developed yet, it may be a long time before a national standard and qualification body emerged
- *National Vocational Qualification (NVQ).* These are primarily skill-based qualifications and currently a module exists for social work and care staff training. It covers how to enable individuals to establish their need for advocacy, how to obtain an advocate, how to act as an advocate on an individual's behalf, and how to assess the effectiveness of advocacy.

Agencies felt it was critical that any development of standards should be done in conjunction with employers. This would ensure that job specifications were developed to similar standards and a stable occupational structure with clear opportunities for skill development and promotions was established. One trainer commented:

> *You don't just need to stack the deck of cards with training courses in an order and then turn that into a salary structure, you talk about what the job content is, and then turn it into a salary structure, and then derive training from there.*

Most agencies agreed that standardising training to meet employer needs and develop a stable occupational structure was much easier to achieve with advocacy providers within the statutory sector, as there was common ground. However, current provision of advocacy is predominantly within the voluntary sector and they need to be involved in any developments from the beginning.

Training agencies consulted felt positive about collaborating to achieve standardisation, but felt that it was key to sort out issues of ownership and funding at the beginning.

References

1. White D, Phillips K and Minns A. *Women from Ethnic Minority Communities: Their Knowledge of and Needs for Health Advocacy Services in East London.* Stoke-on-Trent: Staffordshire University Press, 1999.
2. White V. Health Advocacy in Medicine. London: Royal Hospitals NHS Trust.
3. Grant C and Deane J. *Stating the Obvious – factors which influence the uptake and provision of primary health services for refugees.* London: Lambeth Southwark and Lewisham Health Commission, 1995.
4. White D, Phillips K and Minns A. *Women from Ethnic Minority Communities: Their Knowledge of and Needs for Health Advocacy Services in East London.* Stoke-on-Trent: Staffordshire University Press, 1999.
5. GLACHC, ROTA. *Health Access for Minority Ethnic People in London and Evaluation.* London: GLACHC, 2000.

5. Moving the agenda forward

This section outlines a number of areas that require further development in order to assist the growth of health advocacy services for black and minority ethnic communities. These areas cover improving the funding and commissioning of advocacy, building capacity among advocacy providers, policy development and research, standards, training and networking, and partnerships.

5.1 Developing networks

The need for a mechanism such as a forum or an agency has been widely supported by both providers and funders. A decision about the most appropriate type of structure and process for establishing it needs further discussion. Resources will no doubt be a key deciding factor. The mechanism developed needs to involve small and large advocacy providers as well as facilitators of existing networks. Key functions to be considered include:

1. A mechanism to share good practice and learning among advocacy providers
2. A forum for discussion and debate on key unresolved developmental issues within the field, such as improving awareness and understanding of different philosophical roles and models of advocacy and their relevance and appropriateness to different care settings and communities
3. Ongoing discussion and development of career and training programmes for health advocacy
4. High level debate and lobbying to embed advocacy within mainstream care
5. Long-term funding of advocacy schemes
6. Research, development and effectiveness studies

5.2 Building capacity among advocacy providers

Small voluntary agencies clearly make a significant contribution to the provision of advocacy support to local black and minority ethnic communities. The mapping exercise showed that these agencies are likely to have minimal resources available to them to develop their services and train staff and volunteers. While small agencies provide a vital service and often plug gaps in wider provision, they are unlikely to be able to meet the standards for service delivery or management that are being proposed to achieve a levelling of performance, without targeted support and investment in their infrastructure, services and staff.

5.3 Development: policy and research

While a number of very useful studies have been undertaken on advocacy,[1] their recommendations and lessons have not been widely used in the public sector and their overall impact on the strategic development of advocacy services has been limited. These studies have nevertheless contributed to the necessary literature base that can still be used in further research, study and training.

Research on health advocacy is by no means exhaustive and there are areas where focused action research may be beneficial to the development of certain areas identified within this study. These include training and career development, cost benefit analysis studies, pilot schemes within different communities, and the development of practical templates that suit both small and large providers. The King's Fund (and the London Region) should work with an expert group of advisers, in the absence of a network or lead agency, to agree development priorities and an implementation programme.

The benefit of an action research approach is that it focuses on practical development issues that exist now, from which lessons can be taken and applied immediately during the research process.

There are a number of important policy development issues for local statutory agencies. The promotion and development of advocacy services should be part of an explicit strategy to meet the needs of vulnerable groups. Clarity about what and how local advocacy schemes can be funded or supported should also exist.

A local charter on advocacy should be developed in conjunction with local agencies. This could include:

- the commitments of statutory agencies to work with, support and develop advocacy services

- principles of working with advocates
- local standards for the provision of advocacy
- a local initiative to recruit and train advocates.

A charter could provide a useful way of building on and strengthening local partnerships between statutory and voluntary agencies.

5.4 Improving funding and commissioning of advocacy services

Different models of advocacy exist across London and agencies have highlighted real benefits in providing services from different access points for minority ethnic communities in different parts of the capital. Future development of advocacy services should not be held up by debates about whether to locate services in the statutory or voluntary sectors or whether services should be established as independents or otherwise. What is more important is to develop clear and consistent criteria to ensure that any advocacy service is first and foremost representing the needs, interests and rights of the intended client group, with clear and transparent protocols for the service user if any situation arises that may be a conflict of interest for the provider.

Funders need to offer support for small organisations to make application processes more accessible. The contracts and grants awarded to small refugee organisations need to allow the organisations flexibility to respond to crisis situations without threat of severe financial consequences. Closer collaboration between funding and refugee agencies would help to align funding priorities more closely with the needs of agencies.

A cost benefit analysis of advocacy is essential to highlight long-term 'savings' to care, establish value for money and counteract misconceptions about the 'perceived high cost' of providing versus the 'real value costs' of not providing it.

Funders need to develop safeguards against going for the easy option of cutting the funds of voluntary sector organisations when cuts need to be made locally.

Funders identified the benefit of a pan-London body that could 'broker' services that were not economically viable for individual agencies or boroughs with small language or population groups. This would enable such groups to buy or commission specific services to meet their own level of demand.

Agencies across London provide the majority of their services within primary care settings and have identified this as the biggest area of unmet need, where they encounter the most hostile responses from providers and where negotiating service delivery is the most problematic. The primary care sector currently provides fewer resources for advocacy than the secondary care sector and should be targeted for development of services, raising awareness and improving receptiveness toward advocacy services.

5.5 Partnerships

Improved working relationships between statutory agencies and voluntary sector advocacy providers need to be achieved if clients are to receive effective services. The benefits could include shared good practice, increased access to employment opportunities and improved service delivery.

Users were unanimous in their view that their ideal advocacy would provide them support across all sectors. This view did not only reflect a desire for more convenient services but also users' experiences of poor co-ordination and links between the different statutory agencies that provide services for many vulnerable people. There is an opportunity now for health, social and community care services to develop a cross-sector 'one-stop' model of advocacy service provision. This approach may have advantages in achieving economies of scale, greater co-ordination among services for some of the most vulnerable groups, better links with local communities and better feedback about services.

5.6 Training and raising awareness

Training agencies consulted were very positive about working together to achieve standardised advocacy training across London. However, training development can only be successful if wider development of advocacy is successful. Thus, initiatives for training development need to take place in line with all the other areas mentioned above. Training agencies were very keen to engage with and involve statutory agencies to develop training for advocates within a defined structure for career and employment progression. Advocacy, interpreting and language skills also need to be recognised by employers in terms of career development and remuneration.

In London there will continue to be an ongoing demand for skilled bi-lingual advocacy. Gaps in provision are only being partially met by small black and minority ethnic providers, and affordable bi-lingual advocacy training is currently only being supplied by one training provider. Clearly, this is an area that requires more investment.

5.7 Standards for advocacy

While there was a general consensus that improving and developing standards for advocacy would be beneficial to the organisation and delivery of advocacy services, some agencies raised a legitimate caution against creating too many formal procedures that would be contrary to the ethos of advocacy. Against this backdrop, however, there was a clear case to develop standards that improved the organisation and delivery of services and the performance and behaviour of advocates themselves. These would provide clearer and more objective ways for assessing effectiveness.

Many funders were keen to have clearer criteria to assess the effectiveness of the advocacy schemes they funded. This would need to take account of the smaller and poorly funded agencies that do not have the same resources, and thus cannot be expected to have the same impact, as larger advocacy providers. A useful step for funding agencies would be to identify and agree core elements of effectiveness across London. This would provide:

- funders with a clearer framework for assessing proposals and projects
- advocacy providers with a template and tools to develop appropriate service standards and the flexibility to develop practical methods to improve their service delivery (see Appendix 12).

Figure 5.1: Summary of key actions to develop health advocacy for black and minority ethnic communities

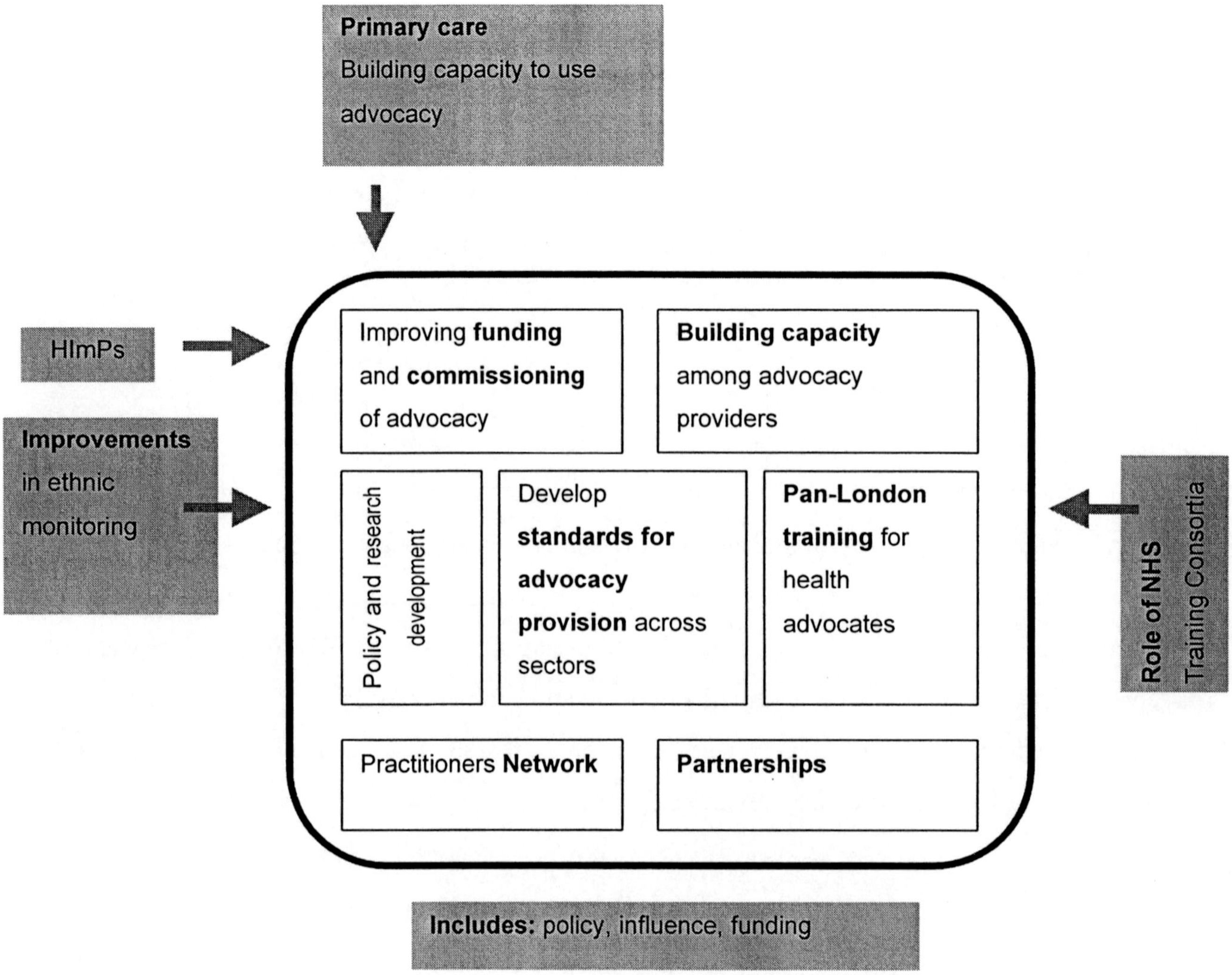

References

1. See, for example White D, Phillips K, Minns A. *Women from Ethnic Minority Communities: Their Knowledge of and Needs for Health Advocacy Services in East London*. Stoke-on-Trent: Staffordshire University Press, 1999; MORI. *Evaluation of bi-lingual health advocacy schemes in East London. Evaluation conducted for East London Consortium*. London: MORI, 1994; Levenson R with Coker N. *The Health of Refugees. A Guide for GPs*. London: King's Fund, 1999; White V. Health Advocacy in Medicine. London: Royal Hospitals NHS Trust.

6. Conclusions

The political environment for public services has undergone significant change over the past three years. The main strategic drive has come from the Government's modernisation programme for health and social care, which espouses fast, fair and convenient services as the key building blocks of the modern public service economy. The Government's strategic policy guidance is explicit about the high value placed on the wishes and demands of users.

This focus has taken the ideals of empowerment, choice, involvement and partnership and placed them in the vocabulary of key policy initiatives. This language is encouraging to many sectors of society, which have lobbied successive governments to take a strategic lead on these issues. Perhaps for the first time in decades many groups that work with marginalised and vulnerable people feel that their interests are finding a place on the Government agenda. The Social Exclusion Unit, the Acheson Report and programmes such as Quality Protects and Sure Start are some examples of where the problems facing disadvantaged communities are being targeted. The Government's compact with the voluntary sector sets down guiding principles on how it should work with this sector. This will contain specific guidance on working with black and minority ethnic voluntary agencies.

While the national agenda creates opportunities for dialogue and change locally, those responsible for the day-to-day planning, management and delivery of services need to be engaged in a process of change that helps them to embrace and reflect the above ideals in their relationships with the communities they serve.

Better understanding

Advocacy clearly offers a vital service to vulnerable communities in London. We have seen that it forms part of the core support that many voluntary agencies provide to local communities. Unfortunately, the manner in which these services are provided and the level of support they receive is not comparable to their efforts and time spent in working with clients to access health services. There are real concerns about the way in which NHS organisations engage and work with these agencies and the support they provide to them. There is clearly an argument that better use of local resources could be achieved through improved understanding of the role of these agencies and greater efforts being made to develop sustainable working relationships and involve them in decision-making and planning processes.

Improved partnerships

The extent to which statutory organisations collaborate to address concerns and developments within the local communities they serve is a situation that both voluntary agencies and users want to see improve. Statutory bodies generally acknowledge this shortcoming and the Government has given specific guidance to NHS bodies.[§§§]

Capacity building

The extent to which black and minority ethnic groups are able to participate in the development and provision of services to the communities they serve is also severely restricted by lack of capacity in relation to organisational and staff development and access to sources of funding. Their relatively smaller size tends to work to their disadvantage and many of these agencies operate at a level well beyond the financial resources they receive. The survey showed 57 per cent of generic providers worked specifically with black and minority ethnic communities and almost half (44 per cent) of these agencies had no paid staff. Capacity building is therefore critical to black and minority ethnic organisations before effective involvement of the nature described above can take place.

Training and development

Linked to organisational capacity is the provision of the advocacy service itself. The level and availability of resources for the development of advocates does not match the importance that we assign to their roles and functions. Across London we found an ad hoc and limited range of services to recruit, train and develop advocates. If we take a step back, we can see this being directly linked to the importance associated with advocacy services. In the public sector

---

[§§§] See, e.g. Department of Health. *Patient and public involvement in the new NHS.* London: DOH, 1999; Department of Health. *Joint Working Between Health And Social Services in PCGs*. London: DoH, 1999

economy we know that the relative importance of services is linked to priority and priority is linked to meeting performance indicators. We therefore need indicators that prioritise the development and provision of high quality advocacy services, with incentives to deliver this.

With the right incentives for strategic training and development, which both advocacy agencies and training providers are calling for, opportunities would be unlocked to create an infrastructure and alliances between training providers, statutory agencies, employers and voluntary organisations to develop better mechanisms to recruit, train and develop advocates. If we make an analogy with a commercial marketing environment, where demand and supply are so closely correlated, the availability and development of advocacy would be a growth area attracting investment and substantial resources because it is linked to high consumer satisfaction and demand. Service providers would ensure that they were able to satisfy this consumer need through skilled and trained suppliers – many of which would be outsourced to the voluntary sector to reflect the niche market they have for this type of service.

Appendix 1

Breakdown of London's black and minority ethnic communities

Black Caribbean

Caribbean communities comprise about 4.4 per cent of London's population. Of these, about 53 per cent were born in the UK. The most concentrated Caribbean communities are found in wards in Brent and Lambeth and one in Haringey.

Borough	*Ward*	*% of total population*
Brent	Roundwood	30.1%
Brent	St Raphaels	26.0%
Brent	Stonebridge	24.1%
Lambeth	Tulse Hill	21.7%
Brent	Carlton	22.2%
Lambeth	Ferndale	21.7%
Brent	Kensal Rise	21.1%
Brent	Harlesden	20.5%
Haringey	Bruce Grove	20.3%
Lambeth	Angel	19.5%

Black African

Black African communities comprise 2.4 per cent of London's population. Of these, about 36 per cent were born in the UK. Africans in London born outside the UK are mainly from Commonwealth countries such as Ghana and Nigeria. Other (refugee) communities came from places such as Ethiopia, Eritrea and Somalia.

Borough	*Ward*	*% of total population*
Southwark	Liddle	26.6%
Lewisham	Evelyn	13.3%
Hackney	King's Park	12.4%
Southwark	Friary	12.2%
Lambeth	Angel	11.8%
Lambeth	Larkhall	11.6%
Lewisham	Marlowe	10.8%
Haringey	Bruce Grove	10.4%
Hackney	Haggerston	10.3%
Lambeth	Ferndale	10.1%

Indian

Indian communities (Gujaratis, Indian, Punjabis, Tamils) comprise about 5.2 per cent of London's population. Of these, about 36 per cent were born in the UK. The most concentrated communities are found in Ealing, followed by Newham, Brent, Harrow and Hounslow.

Borough	*Ward*	*% of total population*
Ealing	Northcote	67.2%
Ealing	Glebe	59.9%
Ealing	Mount Pleasant	56.2%
Newham	Kensington	38.7%
Brent	Wembley Central	37.5%
Harrow	Kenton East	36.5%
Hounslow	Hounslow Heath	35.6%
Ealing	Waxlow	34.9%
Ealing	Dormers Wells	34.7%
Brent	Queensbury	33.7%

Pakistanis

The Pakistani community comprises about 1.3 per cent of London's population. Of these, about 45 per cent were born in the UK. Although they are spread throughout London, most of the capital's Pakistani community lives in east London.

Borough	*Ward*	*% of total population*
Newham	Central	15.2%
Waltham Forest	St James Street	14.2%
Waltham Forest	Hoe Street	13.0%
Waltham Forest	High Street	13.0%
Redbridge	Loxford	12.3%
Newham	Kensington	12.2%
Newham	Monega	12.0%
Barking & Dagenham	Abbey	12.0%
Newham	St Stevens	11.7%
Waltham Forest	Forest	11.4%

Bangladeshi/Bengali

Bangladeshis comprise about 1.3 per cent of London's population. About 45 per cent of this community were born in the UK. London's Bangladeshi community is concentrated in Tower Hamlets.

Borough	*Ward*	*% of total population*
Tower Hamlets	Spitalfields	60.7%
Tower Hamlets	St Mary's	41.5%
Tower Hamlets	St Dunstan's	37.5%
Tower Hamlets	Shadwell	35.5%
Tower Hamlets	St Katherine's	34.9%
Tower Hamlets	Weavers	27.8%
Tower Hamlets	Holy Trinity	24.1%
Tower Hamlets	Redcoat	23.7%
Tower Hamlets	St Peter's	23.0%
Tower Hamlets	Limehouse	19.0%

Chinese

Chinese communities comprise about 0.85 per cent of London's population. Of these, about 26 per cent were born in the UK. The Chinese are distributed across London. However, there are two concentrations – one stretches between Soho and King's Cross, the other is in north Lewisham, around Deptford and north of New Cross.

Borough	*Ward*	*% of total population*
Lewisham	Evelyn	4.4%
Southwark	Liddle	4.3%
Camden	Bloomsbury	3.7%
Tower Hamlets	Blackwall	3.5%
Westminster	West End	3.5%
Camden	King's Cross	3.4%
Greenwich	Ferrier	3.3%
Lewisham	Marlowe	3.3%
Bexley	Thamesmead East	3.2%
Westminster	Church Street	3.1%

Appendix 2

Roles and definitions of advocacy used in developing the study definition of advocacy

Some of the functions and activities that advocates employed to work with black and minority ethnic communities currently undertake include:

Bi-lingual interpreting: undertaken by an interpreter who translates information from one language to another without representing the interests of either party in the communication.

Linkworking: generally undertaken by a bi-/multi-lingual worker who, in addition to interpreting, provides clients with information about available services, assists health professionals and mediates on behalf of clients. Part of their duties is to provide the health education and advice proposed by the health professionals. Linkworkers are often based within GP practices or NHS trusts but are also sometimes are based in voluntary agencies.

Advocacy: in addition to the functions of linkworkers, advocates' principal responsibility is to speak on behalf of their clients and to empower members of ethnic minorities. They relay not only language, but also cultural, religious and social messages about clients to health professionals. They ensure that clients have access to health services, that they are aware of the choices available to them and that their rights are respected. Where necessary, they challenge discrimination and racism and, where appropriate, they will intervene to try to change clinical practice for the benefit of clients.

Community health and community development workers: undertake more generic roles of outreach work within local communities, providing information and advice about how to access and use local services. Development functions often include looking at gaps and options for improving and developing services to meet client groups' needs.

A survey carried out in east London looking at the needs of Asian women summarised advocacy as covering the following range of activities:

- interpreting, supporting and befriending patients
- educating patients to use health services appropriately
- identifying unmet needs and feeding information to managers and service planners
- supporting the work of health care professionals
- working with health promotion services to develop appropriate materials for minority ethnic communities and disadvantaged groups

- meeting clients' needs by referring them to statutory services, such as social services, education and housing, and to appropriate voluntary services, like self-help groups
- supporting clients to articulate their needs
- negotiating/changing the delivery of health services to minority ethnic clients
- providing cultural information to health care professionals and service providers.

Terms used in the report

Advocacy is most commonly associated with the legal profession, in terms of professional pleading in a court of law. The *Oxford English Dictionary* does, however, provide a lay definition of advocate as 'one who pleads for another'. This concept is taken very seriously by advocates and advocacy organisations.

The definitions offered below are used throughout the report. They have emerged as part of the language from the experiences and practices of those involved in providing advocacy across a range of health and social care settings, and are provided to help clarify different approaches to advocacy.

Legal advocacy: representation by legally trained advocates, usually solicitors.

Citizen advocacy: 'refers to the persuasive and supportive activities of trained, selected volunteers and co-ordinating staff working on behalf of those who are disabled/disadvantaged and not in a good position to exercise or defend their rights as citizens. Citizen advocates are persons who are independent of those providing direct services to people with disabilities. Working on a one-to-one basis, they attempt to foster respect for the rights and dignity of those whose interests they represent. This may involve helping to express the individual's concerns and aspirations, obtaining day-to-day social, recreational, health and related services, and providing other practical and emotional support.' This kind of advocacy tends to be more common in the learning disability field than in any other care group. Citizen advocates may themselves be services users.

Formal advocacy. This is a comparatively new term in this country, and usually refers to schemes run by voluntary groups that are not, by and large, user-led. Members of these schemes sometimes refer to themselves as professional advocates. Co-ordinators are salaried and advocates are often paid. They sometimes adopt an 'expert' model of advocacy, which involves them giving advice, prioritising options, counselling and mediation. These activities do not necessarily encourage empowerment through advocacy. They can act for both carers and service users and are often managed by major voluntary service providers.

Peer advocacy: support from advocates who themselves use or have used health services, for example mental health service users. Peer advocates may also be citizen advocates. They may be part of a user-run advocacy group, or a project providing independent advocacy services in mental health units and/or in the community.

Self-advocacy: 'a term used where someone acts on his/her behalf to present their case in a fairly formal manner. It is often used among people with some form of mental or physical disability and refers to those people who are expressing their own needs and concerns and generally taking a more active role in their community. In this context, it is quite often the case that self-advocates from groups to offer mutual support, skill, development.'

Collective or group advocacy: refers to a self-advocacy group or organisation that offers mutual support, skill development and a common call for change. This might include a small group of older people who use local services.

Issue-based or short-term advocacy: also sometimes known as 'crisis advocacy'. This is based on the same principle as citizen advocacy, i.e. on a relationship between a trained volunteer advocate supporting someone who is weak or vulnerable. The advocate is independent of the service provider.

Appendix 3

Summary of target groups for mapping exercise across London and methods used

Method	*Aim*	*Target groups*	*Numbers invited to respond*	*Number of responses, where applicable*
Link agency questionnaire and telephone survey	To provide information to all key people who may have knowledge of and be able to identify actual and potential advocacy providers, funders and training agencies within each London borough/health authority	• Community Health Councils (CHCs) • Race equality councils • All race equality leads in local authorities • All race equality leads in health authorities • All primary care group chief executives • Key umbrella groups in London, i.e. Refugee Council, Confederation of Indian Organisations, London Voluntary Service Council, Greater London Association of CHCs, Association of London Government, Commission for Racial Equality, SIA, co-ordinators of London advocacy provider forums • All voluntary sector umbrella groups	423 sent out for information only, to pass on or refer to relevant providers for mapping	
Advocacy provider questionnaires	To target as broad a range of all potential providers of advocacy services to black and minority ethnic groups in London	• All black and minority ethnic groups known to link agency contacts within each borough • All funded advocacy projects identified by funders • All relevant SRB funded initiatives • All known advocacy	1159 – this included mailing a number of groups twice, as the same people were identified by different link agencies, as well as final 'chase' letters to prompt	163

Method	*Aim*	*Target groups*	*Numbers invited to respond*	*Number of responses, where applicable*
		providers identified by any link agency	responses from non-respondents	
Advocacy funder questionnaires	To target all known and potential funders of advocacy providers	• London Purchasers Forum • All chief executives, directors of public health, quality and commissioning in London health authorities • All local authority and social services department CEOs • All joint finance personnel • All link agencies • All chief executives, directors of quality and business development in London trusts	773	18 (responses not expected from 423 question-naires, as sent to link agencies for information only)
Advocacy training agency questionnaires	To target all known and potential advocacy training providers	• All chief executives, directors of health promotion, personnel and human resources in London health authorities • All chief executives, directors of health promotion, personnel and human resources in London trusts • All link agencies	503	8 (responses not expected from 423 question-naires, as sent to link agencies for information only)
Focus group of main advocacy providers	To explore in more detail key challenges and ways forward to developing, providing and monitoring/evaluat-ing advocacy services with a cross-section of main advocacy providers in London	• All main providers of advocacy services across London were invited to participate in one of two focus group discussions	35 organisations invited	26 organisa-tions partici-pated

Method	*Aim*	*Target groups*	*Numbers invited to respond*	*Number of responses, where applicable*
Focus group of advocacy providers who do not provide advocacy as a main part of their service	To explore in more detail with a cross-section of organisations in London key challenges and ways forward to developing, providing and monitoring/evaluat-ing the advocacy services they provide	• A random geographical sample of providers were selected from the database and invited to two focus group dates	40 organisations invited	9 organisa-tions partici-pated One-to-one follow-up interviews conducted with 4 organ-isations
Trainer focus group	To explore in depth the key issues and challenges identified by training agencies and to discuss strategic ways forward	• All training agencies who expressed an interest were invited	7 training agencies invited	4 training agencies participated
Funder focus group	To explore in depth the key issues and challenges identified by funders and to discuss strategic ways forward	• All funding agencies who expressed an interest were invited	12 funders invited	4 funders participated
Trainer Interviews (telephone and face-to-face interviews)	To capture the views and perspectives of individuals unable to participate in focus group discussions	• Individuals unable to participate in focus group discussions	3	3
Funder Interviews (telephone and face-to-face interviews)	To capture the views and perspectives of individuals unable to participate in focus group discussions	• Individuals unable to participate in focus group discussions	2	2

Appendix 4

The project reference group

Misak Ohanian 020 8992 4621/020 8993 8953	Director Centre for Armenian Information & Advice
Jonathan Coe 020 7630 6111	Co-ordinator Westminster Mental Health Advocacy Project
Farida Malik 020 7363 8132	Health Advocacy Service Manager Newham General Hospital
Pushpa Sisangia 020 8216 4661	Linkworker Manager Barnet General Hospital
Minara Karim 01708 465 059	Ethnic Services Manager Barking Havering & Brentford NHS Trust
Sarah Mudd	Project Co-ordinator – Health Advocates Barts and London NHS Trust
Anne Jensen 020 7247 2944/4429	Making Training Work
Winston Trew	Faculty of Health South Bank University
Nolliag Frost 020 888 04545	Training & Development Manager Citizen Advocacy Information and Training
Ms Anjum Fareed 020 7655 6684	London Ethnic Health Network North Thames Regional Office
Yohannes Fassil 020 7725 3303	Community Liaison & Development Manager KCW Health Authority

Susan Elizabeth 020 7307 2400	Grants Director King's Fund
Naaz Coker 020 7307 2400	Race & Diversity Director King's Fund
Steve Gillam 020 7307 2400	Programme Director, Primary Care King's Fund

Appendix 5

Map of Greater London plotting geographical distribution of agencies that responded to the survey

Number	Borough
1	City of London
2	Barking and Dagenham
3	Barnet
4	Bexley
5	Brent
6	Bromley
7	Camden
8	Croydon
9	Ealing
10	Enfield
11	Greenwich
12	Hackney
13	Hammersmith and Fulham
14	Haringey
15	Harrow
16	Havering
17	Hillingdon
18	Hounslow
19	Islington
20	Kensington and Chelsea
21	Kingston upon Thames
22	Lambeth
23	Lewisham
24	Merton
25	Newham
26	Redbridge
27	Richmond upon Thames
28	Southwark
29	Sutton
30	Tower Hamlets
31	Waltham Forest
32	Wandsworth
33	City of Westminster

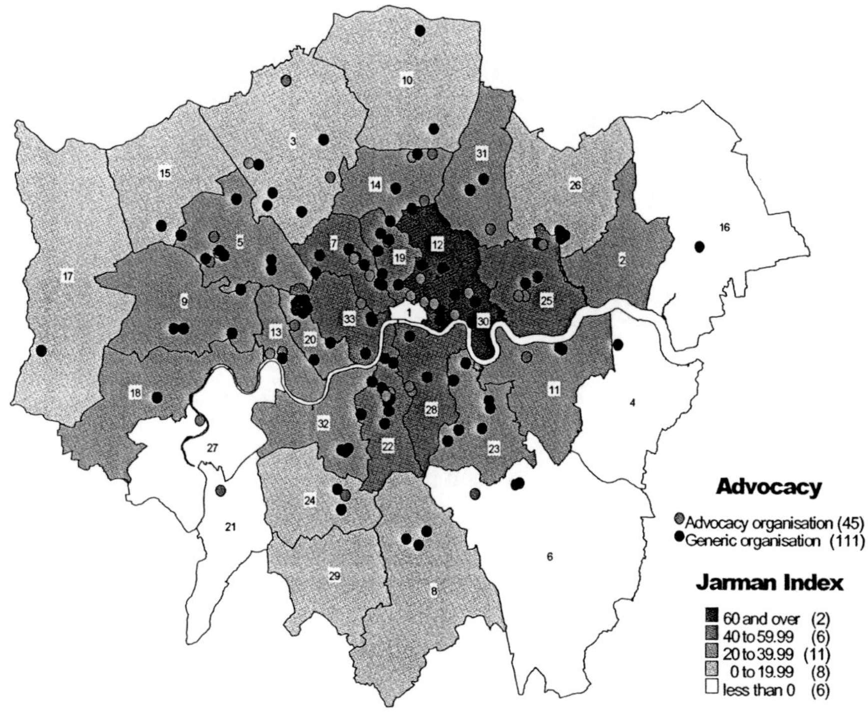

Appendix 6

Provider questionnaire

Health Advocacy Mapping Questionnaire

For the purposes of this study we use the term *health advocacy* to include the following activities:

- helping people to say what their health needs and problems are, e.g. helping someone who cannot speak English to communicate with a health worker
- helping people obtain their rights to health care from GPs, hospitals, hospices, mental health services, dentists, health visitors, community nursing services and so on, e.g. helping someone to be registered with a GP
- representing a person's interests to any agency or individual in the health care system, e.g. accompanying someone on a visit to the hospital
- ensuring people obtain the services and practical support they need to ensure they, or their dependants, are as healthy as they can be, e.g. helping newly arrived refugees understand how to use local health care services.

Health advocacy can take place in many settings: in *hospitals*, in *GP surgeries*, in *community services or organisations*. Health advocates may be *paid* or *unpaid*, and can have a range of titles. Some of the most common are: *health advocate*, *linkworker, bi-lingual worker* or even *interpreter*.

Throughout, our focus is on health advocacy work with *minority ethnic communities*. Research shows that people from minority ethnic communities experience poorer health and more difficulty using services than the rest of the population.

Please bear these definitions in mind when answering the questionnaire.

Remember that any information you give will be treated as confidential.

Please start by providing details of your organisation below.

1. Organisation details

Name:	
Organisation/group:	
Job title:	

Address:	

Post code:		**Telephone:**		**Fax No:**	

2. About the services you provide

2.1. Is health advocacy the main area of your organisation's activity/work?	☐ *Yes* ☐ *No*
2.2. If not, please state what proportion of your organisation's activity is spent on health advocacy.	☐ *10%–20%* ☐ *20%–30%* ☐ *30%–50%*
2.3 Please indicate the type of health advocacy work you do. *Select as many as apply.*	☐ *Helping people to say what their health problems are* ☐ *Helping people obtain their rights to health care* ☐ *Representing a person's interest* ☐ *Ensuring people obtain the services and practical support they need* ☐ *Other (please describe briefly)*
2.4. Please state which minority ethnic and/or refugee communities you provide health advocacy services for.	*Minority ethnic community* (please state) / *Refugee community* (please state)

IF YOU DO NOT PROVIDE SERVICES THAT TARGET BLACK AND MINORITY ETHNIC COMMUNITIES DO NOT COMPLETE THE REST OF THIS QUESTIONNAIRE.

2.5. Which sector/s does your health advocacy service cover? *Tick as many as apply.*	☐ *Primary care, e.g. GPs, community-based clinics* ☐ *Hospitals* ☐ *Social services/community care* ☐ *Other local authority departments* (please state)

	☐ *Voluntary sector* (please state)
2.6. What percentage of your work is with minority ethnic communities? *Please tick the relevant box.*	☐ *0–25%* ☐ *26–50%* ☐ *51–75%* ☐ *76 – 100%*
2.7. Which group/s do/es your health advocacy service cover? *Tick as many as apply.*	*Care group/service area* ☐ *Older people* ☐ *Younger people* ☐ *People who are homeless* ☐ *People with HIV/AIDS* ☐ *Mental health services* ☐ *Physical disability services* ☐ *Learning disability services* ☐ *Ante-natal/midwifery services* ☐ *Other* *People* ☐ *Men* ☐ *Women* ☐ *Children* ☐ *Children & families* ☐ *Carers* ☐ *Other*
2.8. In which borough/s is your health advocacy work based?	
2.9. What is the catchment area of your work?	☐ *Estate* ☐ *Ward* ☐ *One borough* ☐ *More than one borough (please state)* ☐ *Health authority area (please state)* ☐ *Specific hospital trust/s (please state)* ☐ *Specific GP practice/s (please state)* ☐ *Other (please state)*
2.10. How many hours per week is your health advocacy service available? *Please tick as many as apply.*	*Hours per week* ☐ *During office hours (9 a.m. to 5 p.m. Monday to Friday)* ☐ *Weekends (any time Saturday or Sunday)* ☐ *Evenings (after 5 p.m. Monday to Friday)*

2.11. How do users contact your health advocacy service? *Please tick as many as apply.*

Method Of contact	*None*	*Less than 25%*	*25–50%*	*50–75%*	*Over 75%*
Self-referral					
Referred from statutory sector, e.g. by a GP or health worker					
Referred from voluntary sector					
Other (*please describe)*..............................					

2.12. How do you assess the effectiveness of your health advocacy work?
Please select as many as apply from the chart below and indicate how important you think they are? If necessary, please add to the list.

Measure of effectiveness	*Most Important*	*Important*	*Least important*
Informal user feedback			
User surveys			
Complaints			
Feedback from referral agencies			
Feedback from health professionals			
Numbers of clients seen			
Other *(please state)*			
....			

2.13. Please describe or attach any criteria you use to measure effectiveness of your health advocacy work. Please include details of any research you have carried out in this area.

3. About how your health advocacy scheme started

3.1. In which year did your health advocacy service start?

3.2. Why was your health advocacy scheme set up? *Please describe in a short paragraph. Continue on a separate sheet if necessary.*

4. About your funding

4.1 When did you first receive funding for your health advocacy scheme?	
4.2 How long is your health advocacy work funded for?	☐ *0–1yr* ☐ We do not receive any funding. ☐ *1–2yrs* ☐ *2–3yrs* ☐ *Other* (please state)
4.3 What is the total cost of running your health advocacy work each year?	

4.4 Who funds your health advocacy work? *Please tick the appropriate box/es.*

Source of funding	*Currently gives you funding*		*Has given you funding in the past (as far back as 5 years)*
	(please tick)	(please state amount)	(please tick)
Health authority grant			
Joint Finance grant			
NHS trust/s			
Primary care group/s			
Social services grant			
Local government			
Central Government			
Charitable trust			
National Lottery			
Fund-raising events			
Public appeal			
Members			
Private donations			
Other *(please specify)*			

5. Relationships and links with other agencies/initiatives

5.1 Please state whether you have *good, poor* or *no* links with the agencies/initiatives in the table below.

	Not heard of this	*We have good links*	*We have poor links*	*We have no links*
Health authority				
NHS trust				
Primary care group				
GP practice/s				
Health Action Zone				
Health Living Centre				
Community Health Council				
Social services				
New Deal				
Urban re-generation programme				
Council for Voluntary Service				
Citizens Advice Bureaux				
Racial Equality Council				
Community forums *(please state)*				
Local networks *(please state)*				
Umbrella groups *(please state)*				
Other voluntary organisation *(please state)*				
Links with other health advocacy projects *(please state)*				

6. About health advocacy training

6.1. Do you require your health advocates to have any minimum qualifications to work for you?	☐ *Yes* ☐ *No*
6.1.1. If yes, please specify.	
6.2. Do your health advocates receive training while working with you?	☐ *Yes* ☐ *No*

6.2.1 If, yes, **(a),** does this training lead to a qualification or accreditation?	☐ *Yes (please describe)* ☐ *No*
6.2.2. If yes, **(b),** is it provided internally, e.g. from a member of your organisation, or externally, e.g. from a training a provider?	☐ *Internally* ☐ *Externally*
6.3. If the training is provided internally, please briefly describe what it covers.	

6.4. If you use/d an external training provider, please give their contact details.

Name:	
Address:	
Tel No.:	

Continue on the back of the questionnaire if more space is needed.

6.7. What do you think are the main issues for developing and training health advocates? *Please describe in a few short sentences.*	

6.8. Do you know of any examples of good practice in training health advocates for minority ethnic communities? *Please state your reasons why you think this is good practice and supply contact details.*

Example of good practice

Why is it good practice?

Name:

Address:

Tel No.:

Continue on the back of the questionnaire if more space is needed.

7. About the structure of your organisation

7.1 What is the status of your organisation? *Tick all that apply.*

- ☐ *Charity (unregistered)*
- ☐ *Registered charity*
- ☐ *Company*
- ☐ *Company limited by guarantee*
- ☐ *Community/voluntary group*
- ☐ *Self-help group*
- ☐ *NHS trust*
- ☐ *Primary care group*
- ☐ *Health authority*
- ☐ *Social services department*
- ☐ *Housing department*
- ☐ *Voluntary organisation*
- ☐ *Other* (please specify)

7.2 Who is your health advocacy scheme accountable to?	☐ *Independent board of advisors* ☐ *Independent management/executive committee* ☐ *NHS trust advisory group* ☐ *Social services advisory group* ☐ *Voluntary sector advisory group* ☐ *Other* (please specify)

7.3 Who manages the health advocates in your scheme?	☐ *Manager from the voluntary sector – within your organisation* ☐ *Manager from another community organisation or voluntary group* ☐ *Manager in an NHS trust* ☐ *Manager in a health authority* ☐ *Manager in GP practice* ☐ *Manager in a primary care group* ☐ *Manager in another organisation* (please state)

7.4. How are the health advocates supervised and supported? *Please describe.*	

7.5. How many people work for your organisation?

	Number of people	*Average number of hours/whole time equivalents*
Providing health advocacy (paid)		
Providing health advocacy (unpaid)		
Other (paid)		
Other (unpaid)		

8. General issues on health advocacy

We also hope to carry out a number of in-depth interviews following this questionnaire. In addition to the question we have asked below, please comment on any issues that you think we should be exploring further in this study.

8.1. What steps do you think could be taken to develop health advocacy services for minority ethnic communities in London?

8.2. Any other comments?

We want to ensure that as many groups as possible are involved in the project.

If there other organisations/groups who you think we should send this questionnaire to, please write their names and addresses or telephone numbers below (continue on the back of the questionnaire if you need to).

Would you be willing to take part in a focus group to discuss some of these topics in greater detail?	☐ *Yes* ☐ *No*

Thank you for completing this questionnaire.

Please return it in the pre-paid envelope by 5 November 1999.

SILKAP Consultants, 126 Thirlmere Gardens, Wembley HA 8RF
Tel/Fax: 0181 904 8248

Appendix 7

Other activities as described by agencies

Advocacy providers

- Translations – silent advocacy
- Training volunteers to be health advocates
- Training professionals to help them meet the needs of ethnic minorities
- Spiritual counselling, referrals to culturally appropriate services
- Providing health information
- Providing counselling and therapy to ex-patients in their own home
- Identifying health-related issues and organising appropriate services to meet the needs of their client group
- Helping people with diseases understand their affliction
- Healthy cooking demonstrations/health lectures
- Giving information about legal rights and accessing independent information on treatment options for people
- Empowering individuals and communities to self-advocate
- Giving emotional support to clients
- Health promotion sessions
- Training of health workers
- Networking
- Being aware of personnel and health issues

Generic providers

- Accompanying clients to appointments and interpreting for them
- Supporting families
- Identifying needs
- Simply being a friendly face in consultations
- Referring carers to appropriate agencies, e.g. CHCs or health authorities
- Providing information about options
- Producing written material on health promotion
- Organising health seminars
- Providing mental health advocacy
- Making complaints about health services
- Interpreting/translating
- Helping in overcoming related issues, such as poor housing, fear of crime and feeling hopeless

- Helping people question/negotiate community psychiatric assessments and medication levels
- Providing health promotion services
- Offering health education and advising on health issues
- Providing health education via monthly newsletters (not specifically on health)
- Escorting people to doctors/hospital appointments, and providing interpreting/translating services once there
- Ensuring that women receive information to make informed choices
- Ensuring satisfactory discharge planning and procedures for patient and family
- Ensuring that providers deliver services according to their statutory obligations
- Educating target groups in health-related subjects through talks and seminars
- Arranging care packages through joint provision with social services
- Arranging appointments, referring to CHC, completing forms
- Advocating on behalf of the health needs of minority communities

Appendix 8

Measures of effectiveness used by advocacy and generic providers

Type of provider	*Outcome methods described*	*Other methods described*
Advocacy	• Feedback from agencies on outcomes of advocacy • Speed of result • Evidence of the number of users that have accessed the service • Customer satisfaction in evaluations	• Time spent in hospital wards • Review of exit procedure • Repeat use of service • Contractual milestones in service agreements • Review of unit's ability to deal with emergencies • Levels of user participation in the organisation • Number of phone calls received • Ability to respond to new languages
Generic	• User evaluation of outcome achievement • Users feeling more confident even if the outcome is not achieved • Profile of outcome monitoring • User evaluation of results achieved through advocacy intervention • Advocate evaluation of agreement and outcomes achieved • Ability of users to access services • Outcome of contract	• Annual user survey • Use of licensed instruments • Annual comparison of statistics of uptake levels • Verbal feedback critical as clients unable to speak English • Influence on HAZ, HImP and PCG programmes • Responses to newsletters • Periodic case study analysis • Analysis of discharge summaries • Commitment of clients and volunteers to keep to agreed contracts and appointments • Change in services in response to feedback given • Type of use of advocacy and duration of advocacy relationships

Appendix 9

Numbers of providers reporting, good, poor or no links with agencies

Provider type		*Links with…*														
		HAs	NHS trusts	PCG	GP practices	HAZ	Healthy Living Centre	CHC	Social services	New Deal	Urban regeneration	CVS	CAB	Racial Equality Cncl	Community Forums	Local networks
Main	Good links	33	26	15	15	10	9	27	27	4	11	27	19	19	22	23
Main	Poor links	6	4	10	17	11	9	6	4	8	8	3	7	4	2	4
Main	No links	1	3	7	3	6	9	2	5	15	9	4	9	8	5	1
Main	[Blank/not heard of this]	3	10	11	8	16	16	8	7	16	15	9	8	12	14	19
Generic	Good links	67	41	51	54	19	19	44	71	21	25	55	46	52	41	9
Generic	Poor links	21	23	21	26	21	17	15	20	20	18	17	24	18	12	64
Generic	No links	11	22	19	15	27	32	23	5	36	39	18	16	22	12	1
Generic	[Blank/not heard of this]	18	31	26	22	50	49	35	21	40	35	27	31	25	52	39
All	Good links	100	67	66	69	29	28	71	98	25	36	82	65	71	63	32
All	Poor links	27	27	31	43	32	26	21	24	28	26	20	31	22	14	68
All	No links	12	25	26	18	33	41	25	10	51	48	22	25	30	17	2
All	[Blank/not heard of this]	21	41	37	30	66	65	43	28	56	50	36	39	37	66	58

Appendix 10

Funding status of all providers targeted or offering specific services to refugee groups

Refugee communities in London	*Numbers of providers offering specific or targeted services (%)*	*Percentage funded*	*Percentage not funded*
All	23	65%	35%
Any other refugee group	35	71%	29%
Afghan	6	33%	67%
Albanian	8	75%	25%
Algerian	1	100%	0%
Angolan	12	92%	8%
Bulgarian	3	66%	34%
Chilean	1	0%	100%
Chinese	1	100%	0%
Colombian	2	0%	100%
Cypriot	1	100%	0%
Czech & Slovak	5	100%	0%
Ecuadorian	1	0%	100%
Ethiopian (inc. Eritrean)	15	73%	27%
Former USSR (inc. Armenian)	0	0%	0%
Former Yugoslavia (inc. Kosovan and Croatian)	3	100%	0%
Ghanaian	10	90%	10%
Hungarian	0	0%	0%
Iranian	10	50%	50%
Iraqi	8	50%	50%
Kenyan	10	90%	10%
Kurdish	10	70%	30%
Lebanese	1	0%	100%
Liberian	10	90%	10%
Libyan	1	0%	100%
Nigerian	10	90%	10%
Polish	3	100%	0%
Roma (Romany)	1	0%	100%
Romanian	2	100%	0%
Rwandan	10	90%	10%
Sierra Leonean	10	90%	10%
Sinhalese	1	100%	0%
Somali	43	74%	26%
Sudanese	12	92%	8%

Refugee communities in London	*Numbers of providers offering specific or targeted services (%)*	*Percentage funded*	*Percentage not funded*
Syrian	0	0%	0%
Tamil	4	75%	25%
Togolese/Ivorian	8	87%	13%
Turkish	5	80%	20%
Ugandan	13	85%	15%
Zairian (Democratic Republic of Congo)	10	90%	10%

List of groups source: Aldous J, Bardsley M, Daniell R, Gair R, Jacobson B, Lowdell C, Morgan D, Storkey M and Taylor G. *Refugee Health in London*. London: The Health of Londoners Project, 1999.

Appendix 11

Advocacy networks in London

Name of Network	*Aim/focus*	*Membership*	*Specific provision for or focus on BME Issues*	*Future priorities/ areas of work*
Citizen Advocacy Information & Training (Pan-London advocacy network) Established 1994	A resource for citizen advocacy schemes in London and the rest of the UK, providing: • quarterly newsletters • a databank of information • a databank of schemes in the UK to refer people on to • regular training	300 organisations	Currently running project to link citizen advocacy with similar activities in black and minority ethnic communities	• Strategy to link other active 'citizenship'-type activities • Marketing strategy for citizen advocacy • Project to link all advocacy networks across London
Greater London Mental Health Network Established 1995	A forum for advocates to provide, support and exchange information, and to promote good practice and quality in independent mental health advocacy	50 organisations on current mailing list	No – although identified as an issue the forum needs to address	• Training • Providing information • Sharing good practice • Provider support • Campaigning and responding to wider developments
London Advocacy for Older People Network Established 1997	For anyone providing advocacy to older people regardless of the model they use	Not known	No	• Training • Newsletter • Information sharing and learning

Appendix 12

Model for developing criteria to assess impact of advocacy services

Above the line can be regarded as **'added value'** impact criteria for small, low funded organisations.

Below the line would be **'essential'** impact criteria for even the smallest agencies. These can be seen as realistic baseline expectations of funding agencies for small and poorly resourced groups, in terms of monitoring the impact of their work.

Improved social inclusion

In terms of:
Increased confidence
Use of full range of services available

Impact on wider service delivery

Structure
Location
Information
Personnel
Training/skills
Changing patterns of service use

Impact on individual health

Measured and assessed using:
Case studies
Surveys
Easier to access
Improved communication

◄ - ►

Customer satisfaction with the service

Questionnaires
Case studies
Ongoing sampling
Proforma monitoring

Basic data collection re: service use

Define baselines

Statement of service aims

Written information provided to service users

Appendix 13

The role of different bi-lingual workers

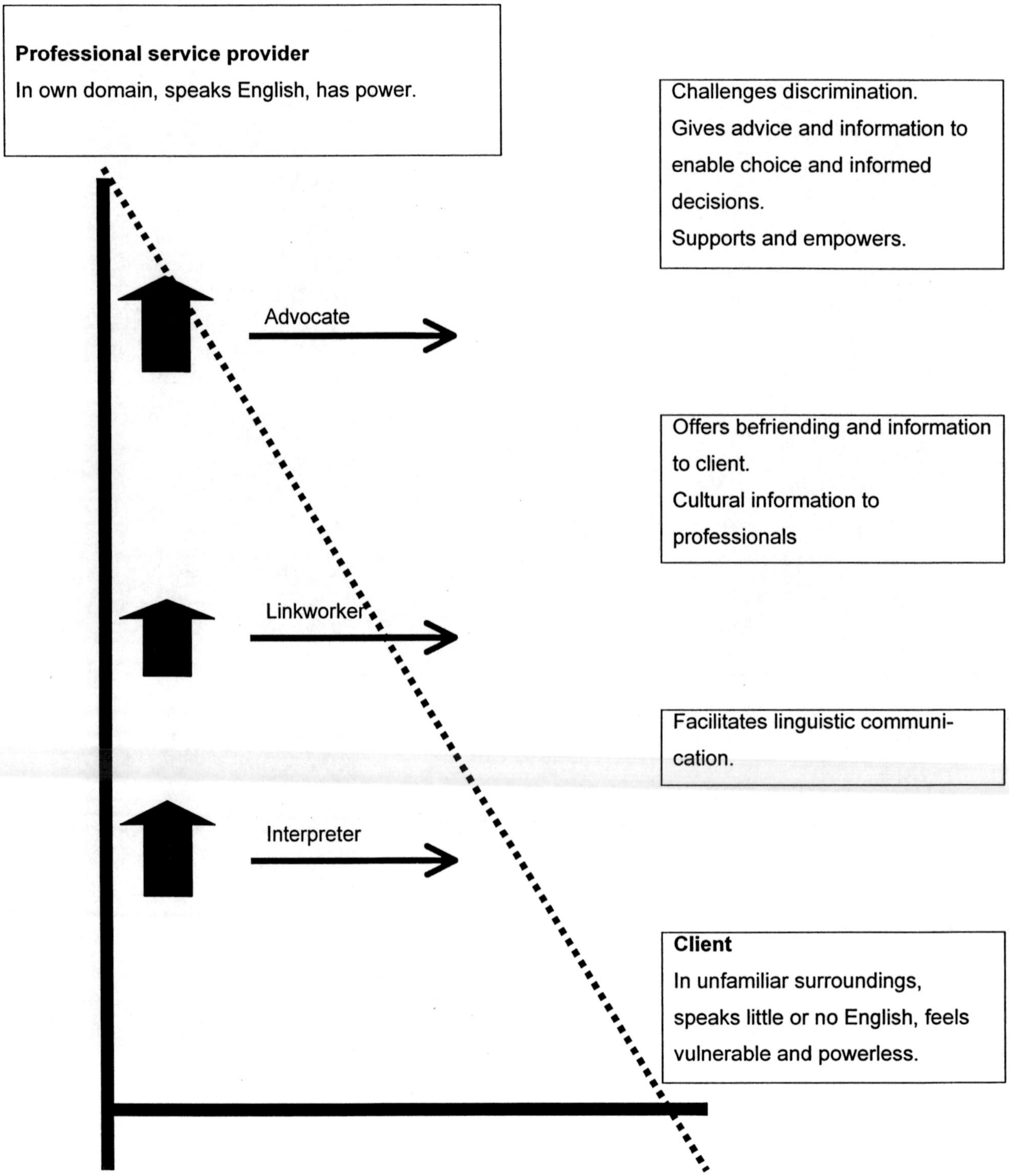

Appendix 14

Good practice from advocacy agencies across London

Local advocacy networks

The Newham Advocacy Consortium involves representatives from different local advocacy services. Groups discuss issues that are important to them such as funding, training, standardising services, developing out-of-hours services, etc.

A support group for advocates was established to encourage many of the small isolated groups that only have one or two and advocates to meet and support each other.

The network is developing and groups are finding it to be very beneficial. Members now share their skills and information about their services on a regular basis. Many members are developing specific skills and building their confidence, for example individuals are starting to take the initiative in running the sessions and setting the agendas, people might organise a session on stress management or how to chair a meeting.

Approaches to advocacy leading to long-term community development

The *Mosaada Centre for Single Women* in London is an independent agency, which tries to stimulate change through group or collective advocacy in institutions, policies and practices. Volunteers are trained as citizen advocates to help and support individuals to move towards self-advocacy through providing structured training programmes for them to develop skills that will help attain longer-term employment.

The Centre organises programmes to help young single unemployed women find employment and avoid the dangers of resorting to prostitution. The programmes also help older women and women who have lived outside London cope with the cultural shock of moving to the capital. They are helped to feel confident and to overcome fears of feeling unsafe and being unable to cope, for example being able to use public transport if they cannot speak English or taking a flat and being able to cope with bills, etc.

The Windmill Centre in Wandsworth provides hands-on advocacy through staff and trained volunteers as well as promoting self-advocacy by providing women, many of whom are recent arrivals into the country, with the likes of computer skills, thereby developing and encouraging women to become more independent.

The Centre aims to promote greater independence and to empower women and their children to participate in society by supporting their emotional, practical and training needs. It provides:

- English language and vocational courses
- nursery provision for children of women attending classes
- short-stay accommodation
- resettlement support and a network for ongoing support.

Capacity building and partnerships

Wandsworth Council undertook a three-year project to improve access to social care services and increase the involvement of black and minority ethnic community organisations as providers of social care services. The project comprised of:

- training for agencies to develop business plans in order to apply for approved provider status
- meetings between organisations and social service care and management staff to clarify understandings and expectations of respective roles and develop working relationships
- development work with individual organisations
- a guidance manual for black and minority ethnic organisations wanting to establish community businesses in the social care sector.

The project enabled six organisations to become *approved providers* social services providers and increased referrals from black and minority ethnic groups.

Targeting needs of refugees in primary care

The *Ravensbourne NHS Trust Primary Care Refugee Project* was set up to provide refugees and their families with appropriate information and advice about the health care system and other services in Bromley. It also has an advocacy and training role, acts as a resource for local primary care teams and fosters links with local voluntary agencies working with refugees.

The Project has developed a practical resource pack for asylum seekers and is working with a local college to provide appropriate English for Speakers of Other Languages (ESOL) classes for their client group. A salaried dentist has been appointed to run open access dental clinics.

Improving access in primary care

In the 1980s and 1990s, *East London and City Health Authority* worked in partnership with the Family Health Services Authority to provide Turkish and

Bengali advocates at the John Scott Centre to support local primary care services. Their experience of using advocates highlighted a marked increase over time in the uptake of services by members of these communities.

Strategic planning and development

East London and City Health Authority under took a review of its health advocacy services, addressing issues of access, equity of provision and consistency of standards as a large proportion of its population had difficulty gaining access to health services.

The results of the review highlighted the additional costs for providing services in areas that had large minority ethnic groups and were sent to Central Government. As a result, the Health Authority received substantial funding. The review's findings have become a useful tool for the Health Authority as part of its longer-term strategy, which will be addressed via a Health Action Zone workstream.

Embedding advocacy in mainstream planning

In *East London and The City*, the Health Action Zone is undertaking work on access and advocacy that includes a 'Charter of Access'. All commissioners of services are now asked to included advocacy as part of the services that are commissioned

While this strategy may not necessarily increase the total amount of money available for advocacy, it focuses attention on advocacy and access.

Training and development for service providers

KCW Health Authority and Westminster Social Services have commissioned an 18-month programme to raise awareness among health, social and community services providers about advocacy, to develop appropriate training for statutory agencies and produce advocacy standards and guidelines. The initiative involves using a participatory action research approach to bring together all local stakeholders in shaping the training and standards to reflect best practice and the needs of staff.

Partnership between statutory and voluntary agencies

The Newham Advocacy Project. In Newham, Health and Social Services made a successful bid for an SRB Advocacy Project. This Project provides capacity building, co-ordination of advocacy services, standard setting and training. The Project Co-ordinator reports to Social Services, together with the Newham Advocacy Steering Group. The Newham Advocacy Consortium provides the forum for partnership working.

The Initiative has developed and agreed standards for advocacy, as well as a training programme to develop core competency skills for advocates, based on the agreed standards. Many participants have used the training as a step to secure employment or to access higher education.

The Project is co-ordinating the development of a National Qualification in Advocacy, which was piloted in September 2000. Access for this qualification includes an accredited community interpreting course, health advocacy course, health and social care access courses. The applicant's qualifications from their country of origin are also taken into account. The focus is to improve services for hard to reach communities and create pathways to higher education and higher socio-economic status for disadvantaged communities.

The Newham Advocacy Project's success is based on a partnership model of developing services that can be replicated in a variety of situations if the partnership is based upon agreed common objectives.